FIRST AID FOR DOGS

"Having read quite a few of this kind of book from a number of approaches (as a veterinarian and as an avid pet owner myself), I can tell you that from both points of view, this book answers all my questions . . . I hope you'll never need it, but if you do, don't worry. All the answers are here."

From the Foreword by
—Seth A. Koch, V.M.D., MMSc.

· HOW TO HANDLE ANY EMERGENCY SITUATION
· HOW TO CARE FOR SICK AND INJURED DOGS
· HOW TO BREED YOUR DOG AND CARE FOR PUPPIES
· HOW TO KEEP YOUR DOG HEALTHY AND IN TOP CONDITION

With more than 75 line drawings, a quick-reference emergency chart and step-by-step instructions, *First Aid for Dogs* is an authoritative and invaluable handbook that can literally save your dog's life.

FIRST AID
FOR DOGS

BY SHIRLEE A. KALSTONE AND
WALTER McNAMARA

Illustrations by Judith Tillinger

BANTAM BOOKS
TORONTO · NEW YORK · LONDON · SYDNEY

FIRST AID FOR DOGS
A Bantam Book

PRINTING HISTORY
Arco edition published August 1980
Bantam edition / April 1983

ISBN 0-553-20196-4

Published simultaneously in the United States and Canada

Bantam Books are published by Bantam Books, Inc. Its
trademark, consisting of the words "Bantam Books" and
the portrayal of a rooster, is Registered in U.S. Patent and
Trademark Office and in other countries. Marca Regis-
trada, Bantam Books, Inc., 666 Fifth Avenue, New York,
New York 10103.

PRINTED IN THE UNITED STATES OF AMERICA

O 0 9 8 7 6 5 4 3 2 1

NOTICE TO READERS

The procedures suggested in this book are considered to be valid and cautious methods of dealing with emergencies and other conditions. The first-aid practices in section I, "Emergency Care of Dogs," are not complete treatments, but only emergency action that you can take to help save a dog's life until a veterinarian can be reached. Your action depends on the type of illness or accident, the extent of injury, and how quickly a veterinarian can be reached. In case of accident or illness, seek veterinary treatment as soon as possible. The authors are not responsible for any loss or damage sustained by following the practices suggested in this book.

EMERGENCY CHART

The chart on the next page lists a number of serious but easy-to-recognize symptoms and a list of emergency conditions that can cause these signs.

When an emergency occurs, you may be confused about what immediate action to take. It may be difficult to know the cause of the emergency, to judge which conditions are serious and require immediate action and which are not critical, and to know what procedures to follow in an emergency.

Remember, while dogs can't tell us what the trouble is, they can show us. Become familiar with the various signs and symptoms; by determining how they are grouped together, you may be able to identify the possible cause, turn quickly to the correct pages in this book, and perform the necessary first aid that can relieve suffering or help save your dog's life until a veterinarian can be reached.

Learn to use the chart carefully and sensibly because, in an emergency, it can be *the most important page in this book.*

EMERGENCY CHART: Symptoms vs. Possible Conditions

Symptom	Abdominal injuries	Allergy	Anaphylactic shock	Respiratory problems	Bleeding	Bloat	Bleeding: internal	Cardiac arrest	Burns: chemical	Chest injuries	Choking	Drug overdose*
Abdominal swelling						•						
Shallow or rapid breathing			•	•		•	•	•				•
Collapse	•		•			•				•	•	
Abdominal pain	•					•						
Loss of consciousness	•			•				•			•	•
Absence of heartbeat or pulse								•				
Dilated eye pupils				•				•				
Cold skin and extremities							•	•				•
Difficulty in breathing		•	•	•				•		•	•	•
Vomiting blood	•						•					
Convulsions			•									•
Nausea or vomiting			•									•
Diarrhea			•									
Itching/skin swelling		•										
Pale or blue mucous membranes				•				•		•		•
Dark or red mucous membranes				•		•						
Deep open wound					•					•		
Profuse bleeding	•				•					•		
Blood in urine/bowel movement							•					
Red or irritated skin		•							•			
Profuse salivation		•				•					•	
Excess urination												
Difficulty in/absence of urine												
Limping												
Paralysis												
Elevated rectal temperature												
Low rectal temperature			•					•				•
Restlessness						•						•
Dizziness												•
Loss of bladder/bowel function												
Weakness								•				
Weak pulse								•				•
Loss of muscular control												•
Rapid pulse/heart rate												
Gagging/trying to vomit											•	
Shock	•					•	•			•		•

Electrical shock

Face and neck emergencies

Foot injuries

Foreign objects swallowed

Fractures, dislocations, etc.

Frostbite or freezing

Head injuries

Heat stroke

Insect bites and stings*

Paralysis

Poisoning: swallowed poisons*

Poisoning: skin contact poisons

Poisoning: inhaled poisons*

Shock

Snakebite

Spinal injuries

Urinary tract emergencies: ruptured bladder

Urinary tract emergencies: cystitis

Urinary tract obstructions: stones

Uterine infections

*Depends on type.

ACKNOWLEDGMENTS

The following veterinarians have contributed their time and expertise in discussing information contained in the various chapters. The authors are especially grateful and acknowledge their contributions:

Bruce S. Ott, D.V.M.

Seth A. Koch, V.M.D., MMSc.

Mark L. Morris, D.V.M., M.S., Ph.D.

The authors would also like to express their appreciation to the following people and organizations for their contributions to First Aid for Dogs: Dr. Henry J. Heimlich, Professor of Advanced Clinical Sciences at Xavier University, Cincinnati, Ohio, inventor of the "Heimlich Maneuver" and Edumed, Inc.; The Morris Animal Foundation of Denver, Colorado for information from their Canine Bloat Panel (and to Jordan Dann, D.V.M. of the panel for his advice) and from Dr. Michael Lorenz's program "Kidney and Urogenital Diseases of Dogs" presented at a Morris Animal Foundation dog health seminar; The Humane Society of the United States; Gretchen Scanlan of the Kent Animal Shelter in Calverton, N.Y.; The University of Pennsylvania School of Veterinary Medicine for permission to include material from their seventh annual symposium.

Grateful acknowledgment is made for permission to quote material from:

Canine Dietetics: Nutritional Management in Health and Disease by Mark L. Morris, Jr., D.V.M., M.S., Ph.D., © 1977 Mark Morris Associates, Topeka, Kansas.

Anorexia: A Commentary on Nutritional Management of Small Animals, by Mark L. Morris, Jr., D.V.M., M.S., Ph.D., and Stanley M. Teeter, B.S., D.V.M., © 1976 Mark Morris Associates, Topeka, Kansas.

FOREWORD

There are lots of adjectives that are used to describe good things . . . "stupendous," "superlative," "fantastic" . . . all of them clichés. But there is no other way to adequately talk about the following pages.

From the beginning, the reader is impressed by the authors' knowledge and the informative approach that they take in putting it all on paper.

Having read quite a few of this kind of book from a number of approaches (as a veterinarian and as an avid pet owner myself), I can tell you that from both points of view, this book answers all my questions.

The sections on "Home Nursing" and "Breeding and Reproduction" are the best I've read. The section on "Emergency Care of Dogs" is superb . . . in this section, "Poisoning" is so complete that every veterinarian in general practice should keep the charts in his or her office.

Enough talking. Read, enjoy, learn, and keep this book on your pet's "night stand." I hope you'll never need it, but if you do, don't worry. All the answers are here.

Seth A. Koch, V.M.D., MMSc.

CONTENTS

Section II
HOME NURSING:
CONVALESCENT CARE OF SICK,
INJURED, AND POSTOPERATIVE DOGS 193

INTRODUCTION

First Aid for Dogs is for people who love and want to better understand and care for their dogs. It contains valuable information for pet owners, experienced breeders, and kennel owners, as well as people who work at pet adoption agencies or humane shelters.

The book provides information on how to keep a dog healthy, how to recognize signs of potential illnesses, and how to give prompt and accurate first aid when an emergency occurs. This book should not be used *in place of* a veterinarian, but *in cooperation with* a veterinarian. While attempts to diagnose or treat an illness should be under the supervision of a veterinarian, the book can help you understand which problems are insignificant and can be solved with little or no medical skill and which conditions are serious and require treatment by a veterinarian. The more knowledge you possess, the better you will be able to recognize symptoms of potential problems, discuss them intelligently with your veterinarian, and perhaps save your dog a great deal of pain and suffering.

The information in *First Aid for Dogs* can be used in two ways: it can help you devise a total health care/preventive medicine plan for your dog, and it can be used when a specific problem develops. The best way to use the book is to read it from cover to cover to increase your general knowledge. This will make you familiar with the four sections; then if a special problem occurs, you will know where to turn the pages for help. It is important to get to know your dog as an individual. Once you understand what is normal, it will be easier to observe the slightest changes in behavior or general conditions that indicate potential trouble.

Section I, "Emergency Care of Dogs," tells about first aid, or the immediate care administered to a dog after an accident or sudden illness. While first aid is not a complete treatment, correct and prompt action can save a dog's life, prevent additional injury, and help relieve suffering until a veterinarian can be reached. You learn how to assemble a first-aid kit, how to transport injured animals, how to restrain dogs; then the emergencies are given in alphabetical order for quick reference. Read all about the given emergency from beginning to end before acting on the advice given.

Section II, "Home Nursing," includes convalescent care of sick, injured, and postoperative dogs. Few dogs do not experience at least one illness during their lifetime requiring nursing care during convalescence. While many illnesses and injuries do not require hospitalization, there may be long periods of convalescence, and how quickly a dog recovers can depend on the quality and consistency of care it receives. Even when hospitalization is necessary, more and more veterinarians believe in releasing a dog as soon as possible after treatment or surgery for home care, since most animals recover faster in familiar surroundings. Section II describes how to choose and equip the convalescent area; sickroom procedures; how to keep a sick dog clean and comfortable; how to feed a sick dog; how to determine temperature, pulse, and respiration; how to administer medicines. It offers guidelines for the use of medications. Home nursing does not require much technical skill, but it does require a combination of consistency, observation, common sense, and tenderness. Whether a dog is sick, injured, or recuperating from an operation, the love, moral support, and competent care you give play an important part in recovery.

Section III, "Breeding and Reproduction," covers all phases of breeding a male and female dog, delivery of the puppies, and postnatal care of mother and puppies. It contains information about the female's reproduction cycle, how to breed, prenatal care, signs of pregnancy, preparations for whelping, signs of labor, what happens during delivery, and postdelivery care up to and including weaning. Because a number of critical situations can develop at this time, information is included about breeding and reproduction problems such as mismating, false pregnancy, difficult deliveries, weak and lifeless puppies, postwhelping complications—with advice on emergency treatment—and the care and feeding of orphan puppies.

Section IV, "Health Care," includes information on

choosing a puppy; selecting a veterinarian; infectious diseases and the necessity of immunization; internal parasites (worms); external parasites (fleas, ticks, lice); common skin problems; grooming and bathing; care of the eyes, ears, nails, and teeth; special care during hot or cold weather; feeding suggestions; and many other subjects that will contribute to your dog's health and happiness.

We have tried to make this book as comprehensive as possible, but don't be intimidated by the amount of detailed information. Many guides for the pet-owning public either oversimplify matters or are written in technical language that is difficult to understand. We have tried to include as much information as possible and present it in simple, everyday language. There may be a lot of material to read but when you need specific information and answers, it's all here!

As soon as possible, remember to take time to fill out the Medical Record chart that opens section IV. It is the best way to record your dog's vital statistics and other information that may be needed instantly in case of illness or accident.

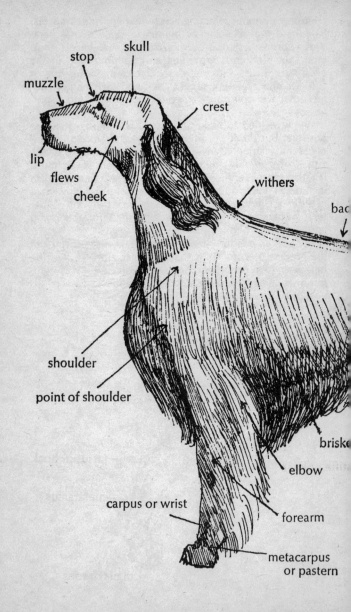

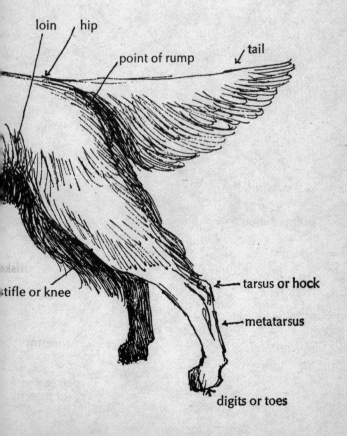

loin hip

point of rump

tail

tarsus **or hock**

metatarsus

tifle or knee

digits or toes

HEALTH CHECKLIST

The best way to safeguard your dog's well-being is to know the signs of good health. Get to know your dog as an individual. Once you understand what is normal, it will be easier to observe slight changes in behavior or general condition that indicate potential trouble. The following are some signs of good health in a dog:

General appearance: The dog should be in good weight—not too fat or too thin. It should be alert, of good disposition, and interested in its surroundings.

Skin: The skin should be smooth and supple, with no signs of disease, excessive dandruff, or external parasites.

Coat: The hair should be glossy with a natural sheen. The coat should not be dry and brittle and there should be no bare spots. While breeds vary somewhat regarding coat, the condition of the hair is a reflection of the dog's general health.

Eyes: The eyes should be clear and bright. There should be no discharge, cloudiness, or oversensitivity to light.

Ears: The ears should be clean and pleasant-smelling. The skin inside the ears should be pale pink. The presence of a small amount of wax is considered normal, but excessive amounts of dark wax or foul-smelling ears are unnatural.

Mouth: The teeth should be white or nearly white. There should be no tartar deposits at the gum line or on the teeth. The gums should be pink and firm, not red, pale pink, gray, blue, or white. The breath should be pleasant-smelling.

Nose: The nose should be cool and moist, with no discharge.

Body openings: All body openings should be healthy and functioning properly, with no abnormal discharges.

Movement: The dog should move smoothly and easily, with no signs of lameness, stiffness, or staggering gait.

DANGER SIGNS

The best way to ensure your dog's good health is to be on the lookout for symptoms of illness. It is not hard to recognize emergencies or serious injuries; however, some symptoms develop gradually, making some illnesses easy to overlook in their early stages. Early diagnosis and treatment of a disease can save your dog a great deal of pain and discomfort. Consult a veterinarian if any of the following symptoms develop:

1. Abnormal behavior, such as sudden lethargy or viciousness
2. Loss of appetite or changes in eating habits
3. Excessive weight loss or gain
4. Abnormal discharges from the eyes, nose, or other body openings
5. Excessive thirst
6. Abnormal swellings or lumps anywhere on the body
7. Difficult, irregular, uncontrolled, or absence of urination or defecation
8. Limping
9. Difficulty getting up or lying down
10. Excessive scratching or shaking of the head
11. Unnatural scratching, biting, or licking any part of the body
12. Loss of hair, bald spots, large amounts of dandruff or scales, or a poor, dull coat
13. Bad breath or excessive tartar deposits at the gum line or on the teeth
14. Open sores
15. Abdominal swelling or pain
16. Difficult breathing
17. Vomiting

FIRST AID
FOR DOGS

Section I

EMERGENCY CARE OF DOGS

LIFE-THREATENING EMERGENCIES

The emergencies covered in this section are arranged in alphabetical order for quick reference. Each subject should be read from beginning to end before acting on the advice given. Particular attention should be paid to the following conditions, as each requires immediate emergency action:

Abdominal injuries (deep) (p. 48)
Allergy: Anaphylactic shock (p. 50)
Serious breathing difficulties (p. 55)
Bloat (p. 67)
Cardiac arrest (p. 75)
Chest injuries (deep) (p. 77)
Consciousness, loss of (p. 82)
Convulsions (continuing or recurrent) (p. 86)
Muscle or skeletal injuries (extensive) (p. 111)
Paralysis (sudden) (p. 133)
Fast Acting Poisoning (p. 134)
Shock (p. 165)
Snakebite (p. 169)
Wounds with massive Bleeding (p. 186)

If you own a dog, there is a good possibility that an emergency—perhaps life-threatening—will occur sooner or later. Animal emergencies do happen, even to the most carefully guarded pet. They don't wait for convenience, and if you are not adequately prepared, a tragedy may occur. Nothing is more heartbreaking than an emergency made worse or a dog's life lost by an owner's incorrect efforts to help.

The purpose of this section is to suggest how to be prepared for certain emergencies. There may be occasions when your veterinarian is not available and this guide will help you determine which conditions are serious and require immediate action, which conditions are not emergencies, what procedures to follow in case of an emergency and what procedures *not* to follow.

If you learn the basics of first aid, if you also learn how

to keep calm and how to act quickly and precisely in a
situation where action and judgment are necessary, you
may help to save your pet's life.

WHAT IS FIRST AID?

First aid is emergency care administered to an animal
after an accident or sudden illness. *First aid is not a complete treatment, but only emergency action until you can
reach a veterinarian.* The principles of emergency treatment are:

1. To preserve the dog's life
2. To prevent additional injury until a veterinarian can
   be reached
3. To relieve suffering and pain

Emergency action must be prompt and accurate, but to
help save a life, the first-aider should learn to avoid these
errors:

1. Improper priorities—too much time spent on minor
   injuries when life-threatening conditions need immediate attention
2. Improper handling and transportation of the injured
   dog
3. Improper bandaging techniques—too tight or too loose

HOW TO USE THE
EMERGENCY SECTION

1. Read through this section as soon as possible and
become familiar with the recommended procedures *before you need to use them.* Become familiar with the
various signs and symptoms. Remember, while dogs can't
tell us what the problem is, they can show us very
specifically.
2. Keep this book where it is readily accessible at all
times.
3. Record the telephone numbers of your veterinarian

and Poison Control Center and other vital medical information on the chart provided at the beginning of section IV.

4. Assemble a first-aid kit in advance. Keep all supplies in a special container and store them in the same location at all times to eliminate the frustration of looking for necessary equipment when an emergency occurs.

5. Recognize your own limitations. *Don't play doctor and try to use first aid as a treatment.* Remember that it is only a step before proper diagnosis and skilled professional treatment by a veterinarian. Even when the problem seems to be insignificant, have the dog checked by a veterinarian. You may have acted quickly and precisely in an emergency, but there may be injury that you are not trained to recognize.

SUMMARY OF PRIORITIES FOR SERIOUS EMERGENCIES

In case of sudden illness or injury, it is important to know which emergencies require immediate attention. In serious emergencies, you may need to act quickly to save the dog's life and know how to provide life support until professional help is available. Sometimes there is no need for urgent care and your actions will involve preventing additional damage, performing necessary first aid, getting professional help, and most of all, offering comfort and reassurance to the dog.

Of course, your actions in an emergency depend on the type of accident or illness, the extent of injury, how quickly a veterinarian can be reached, and the availability of first-aid equipment and supplies. In certain situations, you may have to use common sense and modify what you have learned from this book to face the problem at hand. The following summary suggests how to handle emergencies according to their priority.

1. If necessary, rescue the dog to prevent further injury. Remove from a fire or areas containing noxious fumes if possible; rescue from drowning or from electrical shock or from the scene of an accident if the dog is in the path

of traffic. If rescue is not necessary, *avoid moving the dog if you can.*

2. Maintain an open airway to allow the dog to breathe freely. Remove the collar or anything tight around the neck that could obstruct breathing. Open the mouth and clean out all foreign materials.

3. If breathing has stopped, give artificial respiration. (See "Artificial Respiration."*)

4. If the dog tries to bite, apply the necessary restraint. (See "Handling and Restraint.")

5. Stop or control bleeding or hemorrhaging. (See "Bleeding.")

6. Give first aid for poisoning. (See "Poisoning.")

7. Check the pulse. If you cannot feel the pulse over the femoral artery or detect a heartbeat on the left side of the lower chest wall just behind the elbow (see "Determining Your Dog's Heartbeat and Pulse" in section II), the dog may be in cardiac arrest. Start external heart massage. (See "Cardiac Arrest.")

8. Keep the dog warm by wrapping a blanket, coat, jacket, towel, etc., around its body. If the animal is resting on a cold or damp surface, try to place a covering under the body also, to avoid chilling.

9. Treat for shock, which often follows an accident or injury, if necessary. (See "Shock.")

10. Apply necessary dressings and bandages.

11. Splint fractures and dislocations before moving the dog. (See "Fractures. . . .")

12. Get the dog to a veterinarian as soon as possible after you have completed the necessary steps above. Have someone telephone the veterinarian's office to report that you are en route with an emergency. The person making the call should describe the emergency and give the veterinarian as much information as possible.

13. Avoid unnecessary jarring when the dog is being moved. In certain emergencies, it may be necessary to transport the injured dog on a stretcher or carrying device to prevent further damage. (See "Making an Emergency

* You can find the page number of a cross-reference by looking it up in the Contents. Unless a section number is added to the cross-reference, it is in the same section you are reading. Thus under section I, "Emergency Care of Dogs," in Contents, "Artificial Respiration" is listed as beginning on p. 55.

Stretcher'' and ''Emergency Transportation of Injured Dogs.'')

14. If you are in an unfamiliar neighborhood or another town and do not know a veterinarian, phone the police and ask for the location of the nearest veterinary hospital.

15. Above all, remain calm. Don't let the dog sense any ''panic'' vibrations from you. Speak quietly and reassuringly and stay close beside your dog to offer comfort.

YOUR DOG'S FIRST-AID KIT

We have suggested that a concerned pet owner should read this entire emergency section and become familiar with recommended procedures before needing to use them. While it is important to know how to act quickly and precisely in an emergency, it is also important to have a number of materials and supplies ready for immediate use.

You are at a disadvantage in an emergency without an adequate first-aid kit. Even if it's possible to reach your veterinarian by phone, he or she can give advice but, unfortunately, can't supply the materials you may need desperately at that very moment to relieve your pet's suffering or to prevent further injury. Listed below are supplies that will help treat a number of serious problems.

Instruments

Rectal thermometer: Use to determine your pet's temperature. Use petroleum or lubricating jelly to make insertion easy.

Bandage scissors: Use for cutting bandage and adhesive tape.

Blunt-tipped scissors: Use for cutting hair away from sores and wounds.

Tweezers: Use to remove small objects.

Forceps: An instrument with a locking clamp, used for seizing or grasping a blood vessel.

Materials

Sterile gauze dressings or compresses: You will need assorted dressings, particularly in sizes 3" x 3" and 4" x 4".

A sterile gauze dressing or compress is placed over a wound to cover and protect it from further contamination, to help control bleeding, or to absorb blood or other matter draining from a wound. Nonstick dressings are excellent for emergency use because the veterinarian can redress the injury without pulling away a dried-on compress.

"Sterile" means that the dressing is germfree before use. If prepackaged sterile dressings are not available, a recently washed and ironed handkerchief, napkin, sheet, or pillowcase can be used as a substitute. Should you wish to sterilize substitute dressings at home, the American National Red Cross advises that you "wrap them in aluminum foil and place them in a moderate oven (350°F) for 3 hours, or boil them for 15 minutes and dry them without contamination. For immediate use, a clean cloth pressed with a hot iron or the inner surface of a folded cloth will usually suffice. Do not touch or breathe or cough on the surface of a dressing that is to be placed next to a wound."

Other substitutes for dressings in an emergency include sanitary napkins or several thicknesses of paper towels or facial tissues (spread Vaseline® on any paper dressing before covering a wound). (For directions for applying dressings, see "Bandaging.")

Bandages: A bandage is a strip of material used to keep dressings or splints in place or to support an injury. A bandage should be clean but does not need to be sterile. Bandaging materials are often confused with dressings; remember, the dressing is placed over a wound and the bandage keeps the dressing in place. Some types of bandaging materials include:

Gauze bandage: This is available in rolls 1, 2, or 3 inches wide.

Self-adhesive bandage such as Vetrap®: A disposable, self-adhering elastic wrap that supports tissues and holds sterile dressings in place. Vetrap® adheres only to itself. It does not stick to the dog's hair, so it is painless and

8

safe to remove. When worn, it does not slip or sag. Once applied, self-adhesive bandage eliminates the need for clasps, fasteners, or adhesive tape.

Triangular bandage, preferably made of white muslin: A freshly laundered old sheet or tablecloth also can be used. Make a triangular bandage by diagonally folding a large (30 to 40 inches) square of muslin and then cutting along the folded line. Because of differences in breed size, various lengths of triangular bandages should be on hand. A triangular bandage will (1) support dressings on various parts of the body; (2) fold to form a thick pad, use as a pressure bandage to control bleeding; (3) fold as a cravat, use as a tourniquet; and (4) fold as a cravat, use to apply splints to a dog's leg.

Binders: Use for certain wounds of the abdomen and chest, large pieces of sheets or cloth can be used as binders. (See "Bandaging" for how to make and apply binders.)

Adhesive tape: Use to hold dressings or gauge bandage in place.

Cotton: Use as packing for a pressure bandage or to pad a splint. Cotton should not be used directly over an open wound because of the difficulty in removing the fibers later.

Cotton balls/cotton swabs: Use for applying ointments, swabbing wounds, cleaning ears, etc.

Antiseptic wipes: Use for cleaning local areas subject to infection.

Throat sticks: Use as a medical swab and for emergency splints.

Instant cold compress: Use as a cold source when ice is not available. Instant cold packs may be used for emergency treatment of heat prostration and treatment for initial phases of burns, bleeding, sprains, snakebite, and insect bites. A disposable instant cold pack is a must for a first-aid kit. It needs no prechilling, no special storage, and can be activated just before being used.

Instant hot compress: Use to help treat mastitis and as a secondary treatment of sprains and strains. It is also an emergency heat source to prevent and treat rapid loss of body heat. A disposable instant hot pack needs no preheating, no special storage, and can be activated just before being used.

9

Medications

3% Hydrogen Peroxide: Use for cleansing wounds.

Antiseptic for minor cuts, such as tincture of Merthiolate, Providone-Iodine, or similar preparation.

Coagulant for minor cuts, such as styptic powder.

Mild laxative, such as Milk of Magnesia.

Disposable enema: Use for the relief of constipation.

Antidiarrhea tablets or liquid, such as Kaopectate® Pepto-Bismol®, or Donnagel®: Use to stop or reduce simple diarrhea.

Motion sickness tablets: Use to prevent car, air, or boat motion sickness.

Insect sting relief: Use to soothe and reduce the pain and swelling of insect stings.

Tincture of green soap or other germicidal soap: Use for cleaning and disinfecting wounds.

Eyewash solution: Use to flush the eyes when necessary.

Sterile ophthalmic ointment, such as Boric Acid 5% ointment.

First-aid cream or antiseptic/antibacterial skin ointment: Use as a topical antiseptic for surface wounds such as minor burns, cuts, abrasions, and scratches. First-aid creams for dogs are available at most pet stores. Examples of antibacterial/antiseptic skin ointments include Bacitracin ointment and Dibucaine ointment.

Vaseline® or lubricating jelly: Use under a dressing to keep a compress from drying on wounds. Also use as a lubricant for a thermometer.

Activated charcoal tablets or powder: Use as an antidote for poisons to absorb toxic materials when a specific antidote is not available. (See "Poisoning.") Also use to help control flatulence.

Emetic to induce vomiting: A number of ordinary household products (Hydrogen Peroxide, salt, mustard powder) may be used to induce vomiting in case of poisoning or upset stomach. (See "Poisoning.")

Aspirin: Use to help reduce fever and pain. Give Aspirin to dogs in food or with milk, *never on an empty stomach*. Dosage: 0.15 to 1.0 gram every 12 hours, depending on body weight. If your dog balks at taking pills, a liquid form of Aspirin for infants called Liquiprin can be used.

You may wish to purchase a preassembled kit designed for pet owners or breeders, such as the one described below. For information on various first-aid kits for animals, write Petkit, P.O. Box B, North Chelmsford, MA 01863.

The contents of the Petkit have been selected to provide you with the basic materials and medications appropriate for animal use; it includes the smaller sizes and items not readily available at your local pharmacy or found around the home:

1 gauze bandage, 1" roll	1 Hydrogen Peroxide, 1 oz.
2 gauze pads, 4" x 4"	1 medicated soap, 1 oz.
2 nonstick pads, 2" x 3"	1 medicated wash, 1 oz.
2 gauze pads, 2" x 2"	1 Providone-Iodine packet
1 Vetrap®, 2"	2 Antiseptic wipes
1 instant cold pack	1 first-aid cream (animal)
1 Vaseline® packet	1 styptic powder
1 plastic forceps	1 activated charcoal packet
1 pair scissors	1 instruction booklet
3 throat sticks	1 storage box

Be sure to keep your first-aid kit fully stocked and replace supplies as they are used. If you do not purchase a preassembled kit and buy your own supplies, keep everything in a special container such as a cosmetic case, or tool- or tackle box. Always store your first-aid kit in the same location at all times (make sure every family member knows where to find it) to eliminate the frustration of looking for the necessary equipment when an emergency occurs.

These materials and supplies will cover most emergencies. Depending on where you live and the type and number of dogs you own, other supplies can be suggested by your veterinarian. Some types of special kits available are an insect sting kit for dogs with severe allergic reactions and a snakebite treatment kit that includes tourniquet, suction tube, and surgical blade.

You can make up a smaller first-aid kit for your car or boat. Depending on where and how you travel with your pet, your veterinarian may recommend adding an insecticide, antihistamine, or other medication to your supplies. If a family vacation with the dog will include special activities such as swimming, boating, and camping, remember that your dog may be exposed to hazards such as drowning, heatstroke, snakebite, insect bites and stings, foot injuries, fishhooks, porcupine quills, skunk spray, and frostbite. Consider the activities planned beforehand and be prepared for any emergencies.

Although the subject of pet medicines is covered more fully in section II, "Home Nursing," this is an appropriate place to add a few comments about anthropomorphism, which means "ascribing human form or attributes to a being not human." Today there is a tendency for people to treat their pets—especially dogs and cats—as though they were human. We have listed certain nonprescription medications for a first-aid kit, but we want to add that too many owners give human medicines indiscriminately to their pets, assuming that if a drug is effective in treating *Homo sapiens* it can be given safely to other species. Dogs (and cats, too) often have to take "people" medicine but the incorrect use of certain human medications can be dangerous. Even Aspirin can cause a reaction in certain pets. Most but not all dogs can tolerate aspirin and it is frequently prescribed to help reduce fever or to relieve painful arthritic or rheumatic conditions. However, it can be *extremely toxic* to cats and misuse can cause weakness, vomiting, convulsions, and even death. Part of being a concerned pet owner is learning to treat pets correctly, as dogs or cats, and not as children. Don't give drugs that have not been prescribed or sanctioned by your veterinarian.

MAKING AN
EMERGENCY STRETCHER

In certain emergencies, especially those involving injuries to the spine, head, chest, abdomen, or legs, it may be necessary to transport an injured dog on a stretcher or carrying device to prevent further damage. Emergency victims usually are in great pain and, although a dog will assume the position which is least painful, lifting or moving it (especially a large or heavy breed) will not be easy.

When a carrying device is necessary to support the dog's body during transfer to a veterinary hospital, you

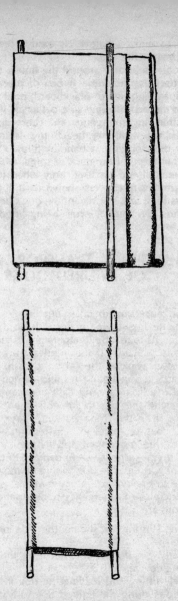

1. EMERGENCY STRETCHER

will have to make whatever is easily accessible into an emergency stretcher.

Many objects in and around the house can be used as carrying devices, including a board, piece of plywood, table pad, ironing board, blackboard, pool float, or heavy cardboard carton with one side cut away. If none of these are available, an emergency stretcher can be made by using blankets, clothing, beach towels, or rugs folded over two mop or broom handles (Illus. 1). If there is a suspected fracture of the neck or spine, a blanket or other soft material should be used only when it is made into an emergency stretcher as shown or if it can be pulled onto something firm to prevent the dog's body from bending, twisting, or sagging when being lifted.

EMERGENCY TRANSPORTATION OF INJURED DOGS

When it is necessary to take your dog to a veterinarian, the technique for moving it depends on the extent of its injuries, on its size and temperament, and on whether assistance is available. If the injuries are not serious, the dog can often walk to the car on a leash, be lifted carefully and cradled in your arms and carried to the car, or be placed inside a carrying case and carried to the car.

Once inside the car, if the dog is not in a traveling case, place it on the front seat and cover the body with a blanket, coat, or towel to help restrain and immobilize the dog during movement and to minimize the danger of shock. *If you suspect severe damage to the head, neck, chest, spine, or legs, the dog should be moved on a carrying device to prevent additional injury.*

The principles of emergency transportation of seriously injured dogs are:

1. Correctly lifting or sliding the dog onto a carrying device
2. Correctly positioning and securing the body on the carrying device
3. Properly lifting and loading the dog into a vehicle
4. Safely delivering the injured dog to a veterinarian for treatment

Additional damage can be done by careless or improper movement or transportation. The dog should not be lifted or moved until life-threatening problems such as occluded airway, massive bleeding, respiratory distress or failure, and shock are attended to, severe wounds are dressed and bandaged, and broken bones are splinted.

Transporting a Seriously Injured Dog (With Assistance)

1. Careful handling is important. An injured dog usually chooses the least painful position. Do not move the dog more than is necessary.

2. If the dog tries to bite, carefully restrain the head by tying a soft safety muzzle around the mouth. (See "Handling and Restraint.") When you handle a seriously injured dog, restraint should be used only when necessary and should be as gentle as possible. Don't cause additional upset to a frightened dog by applying excessive restraint.

3. Great care must be taken when you move a seriously injured dog to keep its body as straight as possible at all times. *Do not twist or bend the body when slipping support underneath.* Use the following steps to transfer the dog onto a carrying device:

Large breed: As the dog lies on its side, place a board or other firm surface of sufficient width parallel to the dog (Ills. 2), under both sets of legs. Assistant(s) should

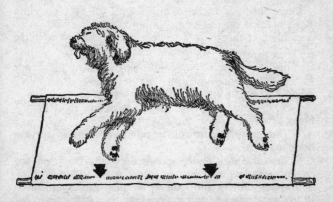

2. TRANSPORTATION OF LARGE BREEDS

grasp hold of the front and back legs and gently and evenly pull the dog, legs first, until the body is squarely centered on the board.

Medium and small breed: Place a board, table pad, or other firm surface of sufficient width parallel to the dog's spine (Illus. 3). Assistant(s) should grasp the loose skin at the back of the neck and on the back and gently and evenly slip the dog, body first, onto the board until it is squarely centered. If you do not have a board or other firm surface, use a heavy cardboard carton of sufficient size: cut away one side and slide the dog into the center.

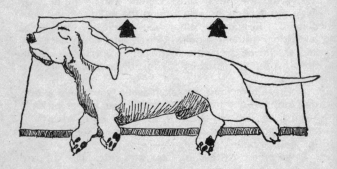

3. TRANSPORTATION OF MEDIUM AND SMALL BREEDS

4. If it is necessary to use a blanket or other soft material, fold or pleat the object, then place it snugly alongside the dog (Illus. 4). Tuck the folds as far under the body as possible, a little at a time. Then have assistants support the body while gently and evenly pulling the folded part through to center the dog. Remember: if you suspect a fracture of the skull, neck, or spine, a soft carrying device must be pulled onto something rigid before being lifted to support the dog's body.

5. Place rolled-up towels or other padding around the body for support.

6. Bind the dog to the carrying device with bandage, straps, nylon, or soft leather leads or any other type of improvised tie to immobilize the body during travel (Illus. 5). Do not tie too tightly, which can obstruct breathing or further aggravate internal injuries.

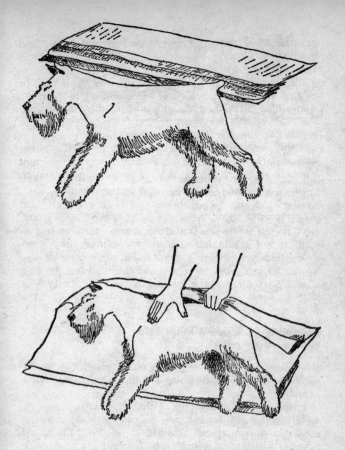

4. HOW TO FOLD DOG IN A BLANKET

7. Lift the carrying device with extreme caution, avoiding unnecessary movement or jarring of the body. One assistant should stand at the dog's head and another at the feet. If you are attempting to lift a large or massive breed, two additional assistants may be necessary, one to stand at each side of the carrying device. Each assistant should face the intended direction of movement and, at a given command, should gently and evenly lift and carry the device to the vehicle.

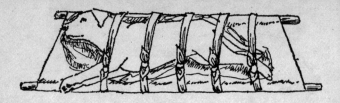

5. BINDING DOG TO CARRYING DEVICE

8. Once the dog is inside the car, cover it with a blanket to preserve its body heat. Proceed to the veterinary hospital at moderate speeds, being careful to stop and start gently at traffic lights. Wherever possible, have an assistant drive the car while you stay close beside your dog to give comfort and gentle reassurance. If you must drive your own seriously injured dog, don't speed or drive recklessly. No matter how well protected and immobilized the dog is, you can aggravate the injuries by pumping the brakes, jolting, or swerving the car.

**Transporting a Seriously Injured Dog
(Without Assistance)**

If assistance is not available to move your dog, follow the procedures described above with the following modifications:

When moving a dog onto a carrying device, it will be necessary to use both hands to pull or slide the dog evenly, always keeping the head in line with the spinal column. Remember: *Keep the back as straight as possible at all times.* Pull or slide the carrying device as close to your car as possible. Carefully lift the dog and place it on the automobile seat.

For dogs of 50 pounds and under, another method of lifting and carrying is to slide the body evenly onto a jacket or coat, fasten the buttons, and lift evenly (Illus. 6), without allowing the middle to sag, or the head and neck to fall forward.

If the dog weighs over 50 pounds and you cannot lift it by yourself, either use a board to improvise a ramp between the ground and car seat and slide the body up the ramp, or call for help.

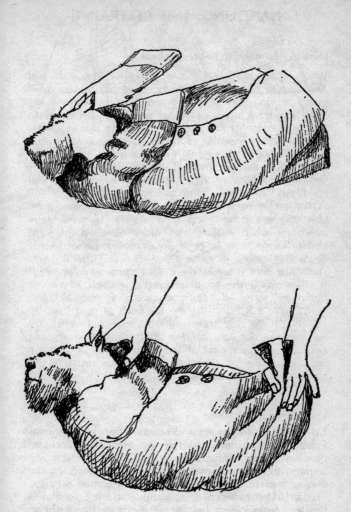

6. WRAPPING AND CARRYING FOR EMERGENCY
TRANSPORTATION WITHOUT ASSISTANCE

19

HANDLING AND RESTRAINT

How to Approach an Injured Animal

When approaching an injured dog, be very cautious. This applies not only to a strange dog but to your own pet. Your dog may be loving and calm, but after it has been injured it may not recognize you and may try to bite. Successful handling depends on being able to understand what is happening in the animal's mind. An injured dog has been frightened by a terrible experience. It may be confused and not know if you caused the incident or will inflict additional pain. Therefore, every move you make must help to comfort and reassure the dog.

Never surprise an injured dog. The animal should be able to see and hear you approach. This is particularly important when dealing with older dogs, whose sight and/or hearing may be poor. Speak confidently and softly to the dog, calling its name if you know it. Generally, you should be able to tell by the dog's attitude at this point if it will permit further handling. *Protect yourself from being bitten* and above all, *keep your face away from the dog.* Next, make a fist and present the back of your hand to the dog. If the dog accepts this advance and sniffs your fist, you can put your hand on its body, without making any abrupt movements. If this is tolerated, tie a safety muzzle or apply the necessary additional restraint and begin emergency treatment.

Capturing a Loose Dog

Dogs that are frightened and in pain often become confused and try to run away from the scene of an accident or injury. When this happens, not even your own dog will respond to voice commands. You must try to catch the dog to prevent additional injury and begin the required first aid. The easiest way to capture a loose, confused dog is to form a leash, belt, or piece of rope into a noose. Slip the noose over the dog's head if you can and carefully tighten it until you have control over the dog. If another person is nearby, a more effective method is to slip two nooses around the dog's neck and gradually tighten and control from either side. Large or vicious dogs may need to be caught by snares or restraining poles. Call your local humane organization for professional help.

How to Make a Safety Muzzle

A safety muzzle is the easiest means of restraint and an absolute necessity when you have to administer first aid. It is important to know how to tie a safety muzzle quickly when handling a stubborn or unmanageable dog. Some dogs will be uncooperative for even the most superficial treatment simply because they know they can get away with it. In this case, tying a safety muzzle will give you more confidence.

Gauze bandage is recommended. In an emergency, bandage may not be handy and you will have to substitute whatever is readily available: a strip of cloth, a man's handkerchief, a nylon stocking, a cloth belt, a nylon or soft leather leash, or a cord or piece of rope.

1. Use gauze bandage 2 or 3 inches wide. Cut a long strip, at least 15 inches long for a medium-sized dog and slightly longer for a larger breed.

2. Form a large loop in the middle of the bandage (Illus. 7).

3. Slip the loop around the dog's mouth just behind its nose with the knot and end ties under the chin (Illus. 8). Then quickly tighten the loop so the dog can't open its mouth.

4. Pull the ends back on each side of the face, under the ears, and tie them together in a bow knot at the base

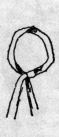
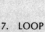
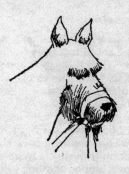

7. LOOP   8. PLACEMENT OF LOOP

21

of the skull (Illus. 9). A bow-knot closing is suggested for quick release in case the dog starts to vomit, because if the muzzle is not released at once, the dog may choke.

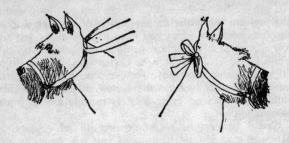

9. BOW KNOT

For short-nosed breeds (Pekingese, Shih Tzu, Pugs, Boxers, Bulldogs, Boston Terriers, etc.) the tie around the nose should not interfere with breathing. Complete steps 1 to 4 as previously described, then:

5. To relieve pressure of the nose loop on the nasal passages, after tying both ends behind the dog's head, bring one end down the middle of the face and slip it under the loop around the nose (Illus. 10(a)).

6. Bring it back to the base of the skull and tie it to the remaining end in a bow knot (Illus. 10(b)).

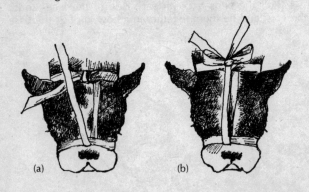

(a)   (b)

10. NOSE LOOP FOR SHORT-NOSED BREEDS

Care should be taken that the dog's nose and mouth are clear to allow the proper passage of air. The dog should be comforted, and discouraged from pulling off the muzzle with its paws. Since a dog perspires through its tongue, leave the safety muzzle tied just long enough to perform the necessary first aid, then remove it.

Lifting and Carrying Dogs

If you suspect a serious injury of the head, neck, back, spine, or fracture of a leg, the dog should not be lifted and carried. (See "Emergency Transportation of Injured Dogs.")

Small Dogs

1. Kneel down and place one arm around and under the dog's body with your fingers in between the front legs to support the chest.

2. If the dog is wearing a leash, grasp it with your opposite hand and carefully tighten it to keep the dog from moving its head suddenly and biting you.

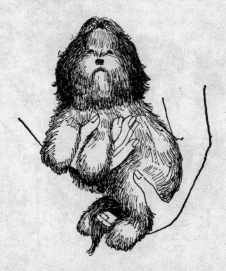

11. CARRYING A SMALL DOG

3. If the dog is not wearing a leash or collar, place your opposite hand at the back of the neck for support.

4. Lift the dog with its body braced against your hip for additional support.

5. Once lifted, cradle the dog in your arms with one hand under its chest and the other supporting the back legs to carry it (Illus. 11).

6. If you have difficulty lifting a small nasty dog, drop a blanket or towel over the dog and then lift it.

Medium-Sized Dogs

1. Muzzle the dog, if necessary, to avoid being bitten.

2. Stoop and pick up the dog with your arms supporting the tops of the legs (Illus. 12). As you lift the dog, hold it close to you for support.

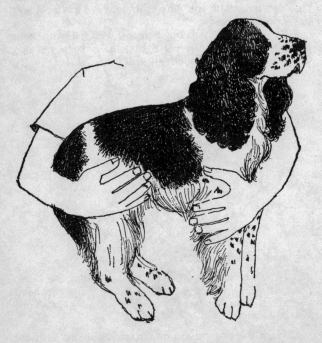

12. CARRYING A MEDIUM-SIZED DOG

Large Dogs

Use basically the same method as that for a medium-sized dog, but place one arm under the chest and the other arm under the abdomen in a sort of forklift position (Illus. 13), for better support.

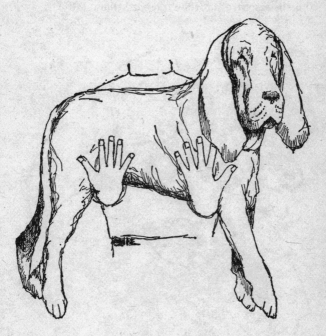

13.   CARRYING A LARGE DOG

Restraining the Head

If it is necessary to examine or treat areas of the head, wrap a towel or blanket around the dog, leaving its head uncovered. If an assistant is available, two other positions may be helpful:

1. Place the dog on a firm surface. Have the assistant stand at the dog's side and hold the collar or loose skin

around the neck (Illus. 14(a)). For extra control, the assistant can steady the dog's body against his or her chest.

2. Have the assistant stand at the dog's side and give support from behind by placing one hand on each side of the head. The palms of each hand should be placed below the ears, with fingers encircling the throat and thumbs resting against the forehead (Illus. 14(b)).

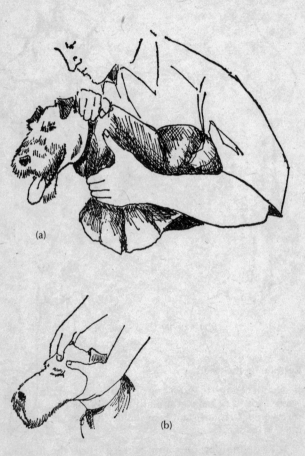

(a)

(b)

14. RESTRAINING THE HEAD

Restraining a Dog on Its Side

It may be necessary for another person to hold your dog on its side on a table while you inspect the body or legs.

1. Place the dog on a firm surface with the assistant standing behind it. If the dog is difficult to turn on its side,

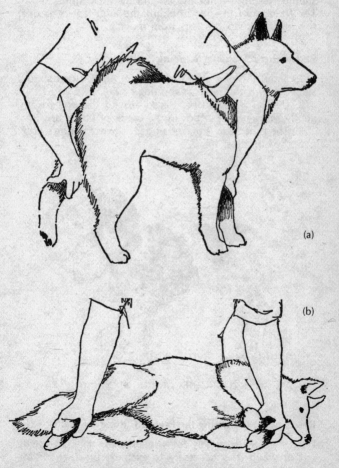

(a)

(b)

15. RESTRAINING A DOG ON ITS SIDE

27

the assistant should hold the front and hind leg (Illus. 15(a)), support the dog's weight against his or her body, and gently turn the animal on its side.

2. Once the dog is lying on its side, the assistant should hold its two front legs in one hand and the two hind legs in the other.

3. The forearm of the hand holding the front legs should rest on the neck to control the head (Illus. 15(b)). The forearm of the hand holding the hind legs rests over the hips to keep the legs from moving.

Restraining a Dog in a Standing Position

1. Stand the dog on a firm surface. An assistant should stand behind the table at the dog's side.

2. One arm should be placed around the dog's front, gently restraining its neck in the crook of the arm.

3. The other arm is placed under or over the dog's body near the hip (Illus. 16).

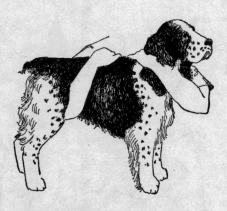

16.   RESTRAINING A DOG STANDING

Restraint for Examining the Feet or Cutting the Nails

Dogs can be extremely fussy when their nails are being cut or when it is necessary to examine the feet for the presence of a foreign object.

1. Sit the dog on a firm surface, facing you.

2. Have an assistant stand at the dog's side and place the palm of one hand under the dog's chin to control its head.

3. The assistant's other hand grasps the elbow at the front leg (Illus. 17) or the hock joint at the back leg (Illus. 18) and gently extends it forward.

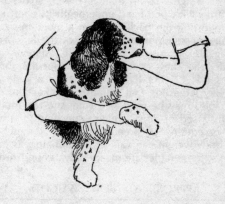

17. RESTRAINING A FRONT LEG

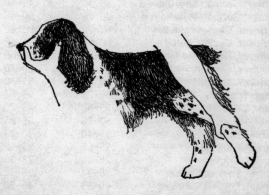

18. RESTRAINING A BACK LEG

HOW TO WEIGH YOUR DOG

It is sometimes necessary to know your dog's correct weight to determine how much medicine to administer. To weigh your dog, use an ordinary household scale. Weigh yourself first, then pick up the dog and weigh yourself again. The difference between the two weights is your dog's weight. To lift a small breed, cradle the dog in your arms with one hand underneath its chest and the other supporting the back legs. Lift a medium-sized dog with your arms supporting the tops of the legs. To lift a large dog, use your arms in a forklift fashion, with one arm under the chest and the other under the abdomen. (See Illus. 11, 12, 13.) If you don't have a scale or you have a very large dog that cannot be picked up, the following tables may be used as a guideline for adult dogs. (They are based on ideal weights specified in American, English, or continental breed standards.) Remember that a dog's body weight can vary proportionately as much as a human's; these tables are meant only as approximations.

APPROXIMATE BODY WEIGHTS

	Male (lbs.)	Female (lbs.)
Sporting breeds:		
Pointer	55–75	46–65
Pointer, German Shorthaired	55–70	45–60
Pointer, German Wirehaired	60–75	50–60
Retriever, Chesapeake Bay	65–75	55–65
Retriever, Curly-Coated	60–65	55–60
Retriever, Flat-coated	60–70	55–60
Retriever, Golden	65–70	60–70
Retriever, Labrador	60–75	55–70
Setter, English	60–70	55–62
Setter, Gordon	55–80	45–70
Setter, Irish	60–75	55–65
Spaniel, Brittany	35–40	30–35
Spaniel, Clumber	55–65	35–50
Spaniel, Cocker	25–28	23–26
Spaniel, English Cocker	28–34	26–32
Spaniel, English Springer	49–55	46–50
Spaniel, Irish Water	55–65	45–58

	Male (lbs.)	Female (lbs.)
Spaniel, Sussex	40–45	35–40
Spaniel, Welsh Springer	40–45	35–40
Vizsla	50–60	45–55
Weimaraner	55–65	45–55
Hound breeds:		
Afghan	about 60	about 50
Basenji	about 24	about 22
Basset Hound	45–50	40–45
Beagle (13")	18–23	15–20
Beagle (15")	20–28	18–25
Black and Tan Coonhound	65–80	50–65
Bloodhound	90–110	80–100
Borzoi	75–105	55–85
Dachshund, Miniature	8–9	7–8
Dachshund, Standard	20–25	18–20
Foxhound, American	55–60	45–50
Foxhound, English	65–70	55–60
Greyhound	65–70	60–65
Harrier	50–55	45–50
Irish Wolfhound	120–150	105–130
Norwegian Elkhound	about 55	about 48
Otter Hound	75–115	65–100
Rhodesian Ridgeback	75–80	60–68
Saluki	50–60	45–50
Scottish Deerhound	85–110	75–95
Whippet	20–25	20–23
Working breeds:		
Akita	80–90	70–80
Alaskan Malamute	about 85	about 75
Bearded Collie	50–55	45–50
Belgian Malinois	65–75	55–60
Belgian Sheepdog	65–75	55–60
Belgian Tervuren	65–75	55–60
Bernese Mountain Dog	85–110	80–95
Bouvier des Flandres	85–100	75–90
Boxer	60–70	50–60
Briard	80–90	70–80
Bull Mastiff	110–130	100–120
Collie	60–75	55–65

	Male (lbs.)	Female (lbs.)
Doberman Pinscher	65–75	55–65
German Shepherd	75–85	60–70
Great Dane	110–175	110–150
Great Pyrenees	100–125	90–115
Komondor	95–110	80–95
Kuvasz	100–115	70–90
Mastiff	125–175	125–150
Newfoundland	110–160	110–140
Old English Sheepdog	85–100	75–85
Puli	25–35	22–30
Rottweiler	110–125	85–105
St. Bernard	120–190	120–175
Samoyed	50–70	45–55
Shetland Sheepdog	20–25	18–22
Siberian Husky	45–60	35–50
Schnauzer, Giant	65–80	55–65
Schnauzer, Standard	35–40	30–35
Welsh Corgi, Cardigan	22–28	20–26
Welsh Corgi, Pembroke	25–30	20–28
Terriers:		
Airedale Terrier	50–65	45–55
American Staffordshire Terrier	55–65	45–55
Australian Terrier	about 14	about 12
Bedlington Terrier	18–23	17–21
Border Terrier	13–15	11–14
Bull Terrier	40–55	30–45
Cairn Terrier	about 14	about 13
Dandie Dinmont Terrier	20–24	18–22
Fox Terrier (Smooth/Wire)	17–18	16–17
Irish Terrier	about 27	about 25
Kerry Blue Terrier	33–40	30–35
Lakeland Terrier	about 17	about 15
Manchester Terrier	12–22	12–22
Miniature Schnauzer	15–17	13–15
Norwich Terrier	about 12	about 11
Scottish Terrier	19–22	18–21
Sealyham Terrier	23–24	18–22
Skye Terrier	25–30	23–25
Soft-Coated Wheaten Terrier	35–45	30–35

	Male (lbs.)	Female (lbs.)
Staffordshire Bull Terrier	28–38	24–34
Welsh Terrier	19–20	18–19
West Highland White Terrier	15–20	13–18

Toy breeds:

	Male (lbs.)	Female (lbs.)
Affenpinscher	7–8	7–8
Brussels Griffon	8–10	8–10
Cavalier King Charles Spaniel	12–18	12–18
Chihuahua	3–6	3–6
English Toy Spaniel	9–12	9–12
Italian Greyhound	6–10	6–10
Japanese Chin	5–9	5–9
Maltese	4–7	4–7
Manchester, Toy	5–12	5–12
Miniature Pinscher	6–9	6–9
Papillon	5–8	5–8
Pekingese	7–14	7–14
Pomeranian	3–7	3–7
Poodle, Toy	6–10	6–10
Pug	14–18	14–18
Shih Tzu	9–16	9–16
Silky Terrier	8–10	8–10
Yorkshire Terrier	3–7	3–7

Nonsporting breeds:

	Male (lbs.)	Female (lbs.)
Bichon Frise	14–20	12–18
Boston Terrier	15–25	15–25
Bulldog	about 50	about 40
Chow Chow	55–65	48–55
Dalmatian	50–60	45–55
French Bulldog	22–28	22–28
Keeshond	40–50	35–45
Lhasa Apso	18–20	15–18
Poodle, Miniature	15–20	12–18
Poodle, Standard	45–60	40–50
Schipperke	14–18	12–16
Tibetan Terrier	22–30	18–23

Before giving medication to your dog:

1. *Know the dog's correct weight.*
2. *Know the proper dosage for the medication.*

BANDAGING

It is important to have a supply of dressings and bandages on hand for emergency use. Furthermore, it is suggested that every pet owner learn the art of dressing and bandaging the various parts of the dog's body so that the bandage is effective, comfortable—and in particular, that it does not interfere with blood circulation or even obstruct breathing.

The various kinds of dressings and bandages are described in "Your Dog's First-Aid Kit." Before a dressing and bandage are applied, follow instructions carefully for controlling bleeding, cleansing and treating the wound as directed for the given emergency. The dog may be in great pain and may try to bite; therefore, it may be necessary to muzzle or restrain the dog before bandaging the wound. (See "Handling and Restraint.")

How to Apply Dressings

A sterile gauze dressing or pad is placed over a wound to cover and protect it from further contamination, to help control bleeding, or to absorb blood or other matter draining from a wound. When it is possible, sterile dressings should be used. A list of substitute dressings and how to sterilize them will be found in "Your Dog's First-Aid Kit."

When dressing a wound, use a compress 1-2 inches larger than the injury it will cover. Do not touch, breathe on, or cough on the side of the compress that will be placed against the wound. Hold the compress directly over the wound, then bring it down into place. Should the dressing slide off before it is firmly positioned, throw it away and apply a new one, to avoid contamination. Use bandage or tape to hold the dressing in place.

Certain wounds are difficult to bandage and it may be necessary to apply a pressure bandage and hold it in place with your hand. (See "Bleeding.")

How to Apply Bandage

Bandage is woven material used to hold dressings or splints in place or to support an injury. The various types of bandages are described in "Your Dog's First-Aid Kit." The following procedures should be used to apply bandages.

Gauze Roller Bandage

1. Make sure that the bandage is rolled evenly and tightly before it is applied.

2. For better control during application, hold the outside of the roll as close as possible to the patient, unrolling a small amount of bandage at a time. To obtain greater support when covering uneven contours, it may be necessary to twist the bandage.

3. As you roll the bandage, each turn should partly overlap the previous layer.

4. The two most common errors are bandaging too loosely and too tightly. When the bandage is too loose, it cannot hold a dressing in place or provide support, and it may come off. If the bandage is too tight, circulation may be stopped.

5. The bandage should be anchored by tying or with adhesive tape. Pins or clips are not recommended for securing bandage on pets, as they can be bitten off and swallowed.

Self-Adhering Elastic Bandage

Self-adhesive elastic bandage, such as Vetrap®, supports tissues and holds sterile dressings in place. Vetrap® has the advantage of adhering only to itself. It does not stick to the dog's hair, so it is painless and safe to remove. While it is on, self-adhesive bandage does not slip or sag. It conforms to the most difficult areas to bandage without difficult procedures and maintains continuous support. Wrapped around an area, self-adhesive bandage requires no clasps or fasteners; therefore, it cannot come undone through fastener failure.

While details for different applications may vary, five basic steps must be observed when using this type of bandage. This is because Vetrap® is self-adherent, requires a loop to stay, and binds securely after one wrap. It is an elastic wrap that continues to exert the pressure with which it was applied. The same property that makes it support, however, can also make it constrict. Proper application requires that it be applied just tight enough to hold and no tighter. Dogs can't tell us when something is uncomfortable or constricting, so be careful when applying self-adhesive bandage and be observant after it has been applied. It is suggested that bandages be removed after 12 hours and the area rebandaged to ensure that there is no interference with circulation.

1. Unroll slightly more than enough bandage to make the first loop. Allow the bandage to relax.
2. Without stretching the bandage, apply one wrap without any tension and press the overlapped area lightly to keep the end in place.
3. While holding the overlap, unroll enough bandage to make the next wrap. Apply the wrap with the desired tension and press the overlapped areas into place.
4. Continue wrapping with the desired tension until the final wrap.
5. Apply the final wrap without tension and press lightly to keep the end in place. Cut off the excess and rewrap; store unused bandage for later use.

Basic Bandaging Techniques

Spiral turns: These are used most effectively on the dog's lower legs and tail. The turns are made by going around the part, each layer completely or partly overlapping the preceding layer (Illus. 19, 20).

Figure-eight turns: These are suggested for most joints. Start by anchoring the bandage around the injured part.

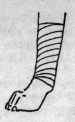

19. SPIRAL TURNS (LEG)

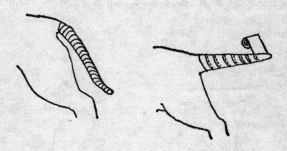

20. SPIRAL TURNS (TAIL); ALTERNATE METHOD

Encircle the part once again, then encircle the area in figure-eight turns (Illus. 21), until the part is covered. Each turn should be uniformly tight; if one layer is tighter than the others, circulation will be impaired.

Recurrent bandage: This is suggested for areas where it is difficult to keep a bandage in place, such as the feet or tail. To apply a recurrent bandage:

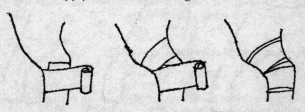

21. FIGURE-EIGHT TURNS, FROM BEGINNING TO END

1. Fold a length of bandage several times and apply it lengthwise on each side of the injured part. If it is being used on the tail, the folds should be long enough to cover the tail from base to base on each side (Illus. 22(a), 22(b)).

2. Make a spiral turn around the part to secure the bandage in place. Then apply simple spiral overlapping turns (Illus. 22(c), 22(d), until the area is sufficiently bandaged.

Spiral turns, figure-eight turns, and recurrent bandage are the types of bandage used in the following instructions.

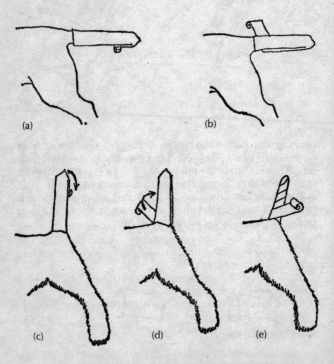

(a)　　　　　　　　　　　(b)

(c)　　　　　(d)　　　　　(e)

22.   RECURRENT BANDAGE

Bandaging the Eye or Head

1. Carefully place a sterile gauze dressing over the affected eye (Illus. 23(a)), or injured part of the face or head.
2. Secure the dressing in place with bandage.
3. Wrap the bandage around the forehead and ears (maintaining regular position) and under the chin (Illus. 23(b)).

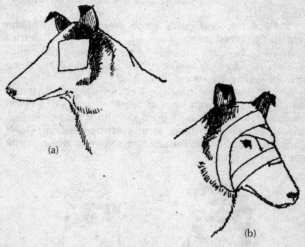

(a)

(b)

23. BANDAGING EYE

4. Because of the head's irregular contours, self-adhesive bandage is recommended. A virtual sphere is bandaged with a flat bandage, but the conformability of self-adhesive bandage permits the dressing to be done without either folds or creases, even around the ears. The elasticity permits the dog to eat, even though a portion of the jaw is bandaged.
5. If self-adhesive bandage is not used, secure the gauze bandage with tape.
6. Be sure the bandage does not obstruct breathing.

Bandaging the Ear

As explained at "Ear Emergencies," injuries to the ear flaps tend to bleed profusely. If the bleeding is severe, use sterile gauze dressings and apply direct pressure over the injury. When the bleeding stops, remember that the injury can be aggravated by the dog's natural tendency to shake its head, so you must steady the injured ear with a firm bandage.

1. Place a sterile gauze dressing on top of the dog's head.

2. Lay the injured earflap back onto the sterile dressing (Illus. 24(a)).

3. Place a second sterile gauze dressing on top of the earflap (Illus. 24(b)).

4. Wrap bandage around the head, leaving the opposite ear free to help keep the bandage in place and keep it from sliding backward (Illus. 24(c)).

5. If self-adhesive bandage was not used, keep gauze bandage in place with strips of adhesive tape. Cut a nylon or men's stocking at both ends and slip it over the head, snood- or helmet-fashion, to protect the bandage. Don't forget to cut a hole in the stocking to permit the opposite ear to hang naturally.

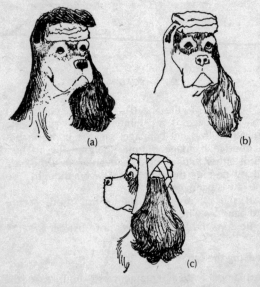

(a)

(b)

(c)

24. BANDAGING EAR

Bandaging the Tail

The tail is difficult to keep bandaged because the dressing can be bitten, pulled, or wagged off without too much difficulty.

1. Apply a dressing over the wound.
2. When bandaging to hold the dressing in place, the entire length of the dog's tail should be wrapped to prevent circulation damage.
3. Use a recurrent bandage. Fold a length of gauze bandage several times and apply it to cover the tail from base to base on each side (Illus. 22).
4. Make a spiral turn around the tail to secure the bandage in place. If possible, push up small amounts of hair and include them in some of the first turns to keep the bandage from slipping. Then wrap the entire tail with overlapping spiral layers (Illus. 25). To make the gauze bandage very secure, you can apply two layers of spiral turns in opposite directions.
5. If you are using self-adhesive bandage, the tail should be wrapped on the loose side to keep circulation from being impaired. This kind of bandage can flex without becoming undone.
6. If gauze bandage is used, hold it in place with strips of adhesive tape. At the base of the tail, extend the tape slightly beyond the bandage onto the hair, if possible, to keep the bandage from slipping off.

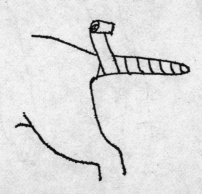

25. BANDAGING TAIL

Bandaging the Foot and Leg

The most common injuries a pet owner faces are injuries to the dog's feet and legs. Even when the wound involves the leg only, the foot should be covered with bandage. A partial wrapping of the leg can create a tourniquetlike effect, shutting off circulation and causing the lower part of the leg to swell.

1. If possible, have an assistant steady the leg to be dressed and bandaged. Muzzle the dog if it tries to bite. (See "Handling and Restraint.")

2. Cover the wound (on the foot or the leg) with a sterile gauze dressing (Illus. 26(a)).

3. Pack small pieces of cotton between the toes and dewclaw to prevent pressure damage (Illus. 26(b)).

4. Wrap a thin layer of cotton or bandage underwrap around the foot for padding (Illus. 26(c)), extending the padding several inches above the foot onto the leg to cover the dressing.

5. Fold several lengths of gauze bandage into a U shape around the leg and foot (Illus. 26(d); see also Illus. 22, for recurrent bandage).

6. The next step in bandaging the foot is to make sure that it is well protected. Use 1- or 2-inch gauze bandage (depending on the size of the dog) or self-adhesive

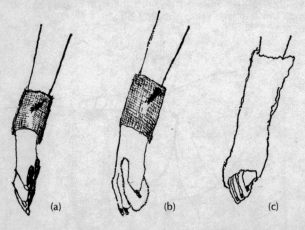

(a)   (b)   (c)

26. BANDAGING FOOT AND LEG

bandage. Start by wrapping the bandage around the toes and under the foot several times (Illus. 26(e)).

7. Work upward, bandaging in spiral turns, partly overlapping each layer over the preceding layer (Illus. 26(f)). Make sure that the bandage is applied firmly—but not tightly enough to stop circulation. When using self-adhesive bandage, the extremities should be wrapped slightly on the loose side to protect the circulation.

8. If the injury is on the leg, keep overlapping the layers of bandage until the area above the wound is covered.

9. If you are using gauze bandage, secure it at the top by splitting and tying the ends together (Illus. 26(g)).

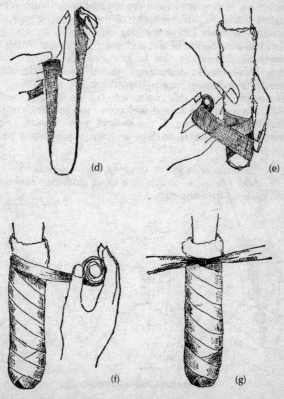

(d)

(e)

(f)

(g)

10. If you are using gauze bandage, wind several strips of 1-inch tape around the bandaged foot and leg for extra protection. Finish with a tape strip that extends slightly beyond the bandage and padding onto the hair, to keep the bandage from slipping.

Bandaging the Chest and Abdomen

Body wounds can be difficult to bandage, but the basic spiral overlapping turns previously described can be used (Illus. 27). If self-adhesive bandage is used, compression dressings of the chest or for rib support are put on a bit more tightly. The conformability of self-adhesive bandage permits the leg to be out of the bandaging, without there being any lumps or folds in the wrappings. Self-adherence ensures that the arrangement of the bandaging will not change, however active the dog may be.

For large wounds of the abdomen or chest, a binder or many-tailed bandage may be effective. This can be made by cutting freshly laundered, strong white material (a sheet, for example) in a pattern (Illus. 28), with strips cut or torn along each side. Be sure to cut the bandage wider than the wounded area it will cover and longer than the body's circumference. If the wound is on the chest, cut out holes for the front legs to keep the bandage from slipping.

1. Place a sterile gauze dressing over the wound.
2. Add a layer of cotton or a clean cloth or towel over the dressing for padding.

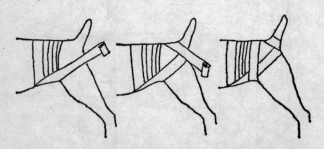

27. BANDAGING THE ABDOMEN

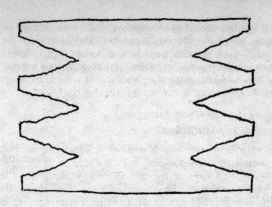

28. MANY-TAILED BANDAGE

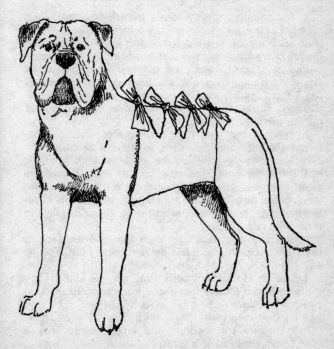

29. MANY-TAILED ABDOMINAL BANDAGING

3. Place the center of the many-tailed bandage over the dressing, draw the material together, and fasten the ties (Illus. 29). Each tie can be adjusted to apply the correct amount of pressure. This type of bandage can be tied along the back to protect an abdominal wound or under the stomach to protect a wound on the back.

Preventing Self-Mutilation

No matter how securely a wound is bandaged or how effectively it is treated, your dog may scratch at its head, face, eyes, and ears or try to bite or lick wounds on its body, legs, and feet. This will not only slow down the healing process, but can cause additional damage. Any of the following procedures will help prevent persistent scratching, biting, licking, and self-mutilation:

1. Temporarily tape the dog's front legs or back legs together at the ankles. Do not use adhesive tape: Scotch® Hair Set Tape or first-aid tapes such as Micropore and Dermicel are kinder to the skin and hair. The legs can be bound temporarily with self-adhesive bandage; unlike tapes which must be peeled off, bandage such as Vetrap® can be cut quickly with scissors and will almost fall off. *Caution:* These are only temporary measures and should not be used for any length of time.

2. Bandage the feet. Pack small pieces of cotton between the toes and dewclaws to prevent pressure. The dewclaw is an extra toe on the inside of each front leg just above the paw. (The dewclaws of many breeds are often removed several days after birth.) Wrap the feet with gauze or self-adhesive bandage (be sure to cover the dewclaw) and remember to secure gauze bandage in place with tape.

3. Slip a baby's sock over each foot and use tape to keep the socks in place and prevent them from slipping off.

4. Use an Elizabethan collar. You may be able to buy a prefabricated Elizabethan collar from a veterinary hospital or pet store or you can make your own:
   a. Cut cardboard (lightweight for a small dog; heavier for medium and large breeds) into a doughnut pattern (Illus. 30).
   b. Cut a V shape from the outside edge to the cen-

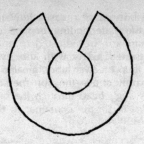

30. ELIZABETHAN COLLAR

ter. Then cut an opening in the center, using the
dog's collar as a size guide.

c. Place the collar around the dog's neck and bring
the edges together. Fasten with staples or punch
several holes on each side of the V and tie the
collar closed with a shoelace or cord.

d. The outside edge of the Elizabethan collar should
be turned forward toward the head and extend
slightly beyond the dog's jaw (Illus. 31).

5. Another method of protection, similar in principle
to the Elizabethan collar:

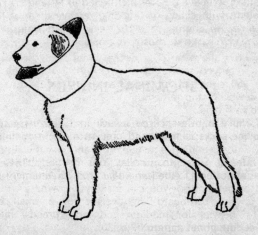

31. PLACEMENT OF ELIZABETHAN COLLAR

a. Cut the bottom of a plastic flowerpot, bucket, or wastebasket, depending on the dog's size and head shape.
b. Cover the cut edges with adhesive tape.
c. Punch four or five holes around the container immediately above the cut opening.
d. Slip the dog's head through the opening and use the holes to tie the container to the collar (Illus. 32).

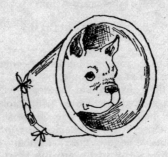

32. FLOWERPOT COLLAR

If the protective devices mentioned in (4) and (5) cause problems with eating or drinking, remove them at feeding time. An alternative is to use a wire muzzle, which can be purchased at most pet stores.

ABDOMINAL INJURIES

Abdominal injuries caused by car accidents or gunshot or other penetrating wounds are serious and sometimes fatal. Extensive injuries may tear the abdominal wall, causing internal organs to emerge from the body. These injuries should be treated *immediately* by a veterinarian.

Symptoms

- Bleeding from wounds.
- Severe pain.

- Rigidity of abdominal muscles.
- Vomiting blood.
- Extensive injuries that tear abdominal wall, making internal organs visible or causing them to protrude from injured area.
- Loss of consciousness.
- Shock.

Materials Required for Emergency Action

Sterile gauze dressings or emergency substitutes
Bandage (or towel or sheet)
Blanket

Emergency Action

1. Keep air passages clear. Loosen the collar or anything tight around the dog's neck that might obstruct breathing.
2. If necessary, restrain the dog by muzzling, but do not apply a muzzle if the dog is vomiting. (See "Handling and Restraint.")
3. If any internal organs protrude from the wound, wet sterile dressings with warm water and cover the organ(s) to maintain moistness. *Do not try to push organs back into place.*
4. Cover the sterile dressings with bandage, towel, or sheet for extra protection.
5. Treat for shock if necessary. (See "Shock.")
6. Do not give food or liquids, as this may aggravate internal injuries.
7. Keep the dog calm and in a level body position.
8. Get to a veterinarian immediately; surgery probably will be necessary. Move the dog with extreme caution. (See "Emergency Transportation of Injured Dogs.")

ALLERGY/ALLERGIC REACTIONS

Allergy is an unusual systemic reaction to a substance which produces no effects in a nonsensitive member of the same species. Allergy can be inherited or acquired.

A dog can be born with or later develop hypersensitivity which causes a reaction when a given material is present on the skin or within the body. An allergy can be acquired when a dog reacts to a previously encountered substance which produced no effects. The first exposure to such a substance does not produce a reaction, but subsequent exposure triggers an allergic reaction.

There are many causes of allergies, including pollens, atmospheric pollutants, insect bites, drugs, vaccines, chemicals, bacteria, food, and mold. Some allergies occur only at certain times of the year while others can occur at any time. The majority of hypersensitivities are not serious and can be successfully diagnosed and treated. Some, however, are severe and should be considered life-threatening.

Two kinds of hypersensitivities require emergency treatment: anaphylactic shock and some allergic reactions.

Anaphylactic Shock

This is an acute, severe reaction in which respiration and circulation may collapse and death can result. It can occur from injections of vaccines, antibiotics, hormones, and tranquilizers, or from repeated blood transfusions, stinging insects, or certain foods.

Symptoms of Anaphylactic Shock

- Vomiting.
- Diarrhea.
- Anxiety/apprehension.
- Low temperature.
- Epileptic-type seizures.
- Collapse.

Emergency Action for Anaphylactic Shock

1. *Get the dog to a veterinarian immediately.* Anaphylaxis requires oxygen and prompt intravenous injection of epinephrine.
2. Keep air passages clear. Loosen the dog's collar or anything tight around the neck that obstructs breathing.

3. Start artificial respiration if the dog is not breathing. (See "Artificial Respiration.")
4. If the dog is having seizures, restrain by wrapping its body with a blanket to prevent further injury en route to the hospital.

Allergic Reactions

These are gradually developing reactions which, depending on the type of allergy, result in the symptoms listed below. They can occur from inhaling plant pollens, skin contact with external irritants, ingestion of foods or other materials, insect bites, drugs, vaccines, or blood transfusions. A majority of dogs suffering from allergic reactions are successfully diagnosed and treated.

Symptoms of Allergic Reactions

* Mild to intense itching.
* Swelling or puffiness of the mouth, eyelids, or other facial areas.
* Breathing difficulties.
* Discharge from eyes.
* Rubbing eyes with paws or on ground.
* Salivation.
* Thickening or lumps on skin in affected areas.

Emergency Action for Allergic Reactions

1. Try to determine and remove the cause if possible.
2. Keep air passages clear. Loosen the collar and anything tight around the dog's neck so that breathing is unobstructed.
3. If breathing stops, start artificial respiration. (See "Artificial Respiration.")
4. If the dog has swallowed spoiled food or other substance, give a mild laxative, such as Milk of Magnesia (2 teaspoons per 10 pounds of body weight), and an enema. (See "How to Give an Enema" in section II.)
5. If the reaction is caused by skin contact, flush the skin with large quantities of warm water. Wash with shampoo and water, rinse thoroughly, and dry.
6. Consult your veterinarian. If the cause of the allergy is not known, diagnosis will involve examination, col-

lecting a history of the dog's symptoms or reactions, and performing laboratory and skin tests.

ANAL GLAND IMPACTION

All dogs have a pair of anal glands situated under the skin at each side of the opening to the rectum (Illus. 33). It's easy to locate these pear-shaped sacs externally by placing your thumb on one side of the anal opening and your index finger on the other side. Some experts believe that the anal glands lubricate the passage of bowel movements. Others think that they are involved in sex determination—that the odor secreted by these glands enables a dog to determine the sex of another dog upon meeting. A third theory is that the anal sacs are vestigal scent glands left over from the dog's primitive state, and that they once functioned like those of a skunk to frighten away possible attackers.

Normally these glands secrete a watery, brownish fluid which empties into the rectum. At times they can become clogged and accumulate a foul-smelling mass inside.

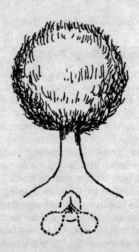

33. ANAL SACS

Often, upon examination, the rectum appears to be inflamed and the sacs may be enlarged, bulging from the retention of accumulated fluid. Anal gland impaction can occur in all breeds, but it seems to be more common in smaller dogs, perhaps because they are fed softer diets. Larger dogs tend to eat bulkier foods, producing stiffer fecal matter which seems to help prevent clogged anal sacs. Impaction of the anal glands can cause considerable pain and discomfort to your dog.

Symptoms

- Frequent licking or biting at the anus.
- Dragging the rear end across the ground.
- Foul smell at the rectal area.
- Irritated anus.
- Listlessness.
- Dull appearance of eyes.
- Constipation (not always present).

Materials Required for Action

Absorbent cotton or antiseptic wipes
First-aid cream

Action

1. Expressing the clogged glands usually will bring relief.
2. Stand the dog on a firm surface. Hold up the tail in one hand.
3. It is necessary to cover the anus with absorbent cotton or an antiseptic wipe, as the accumulation will spurt out when the glands are being emptied.
4. Hold the cotton or wipe in your free hand and place it over the anal opening. Place your thumb on one side of the anus and your index and second fingers on the other side (Illus. 34). Gently squeeze together until the contents of the glands squirt out.
5. Usually the slightest pressure will release the accumulated fluid, but if your dog has glands which are difficult to express, pressure should be exerted in a different way to release the fluid. Try to place your thumb and fingers underneath and slightly behind the glands, then squeeze gently in an upward and outward motion.

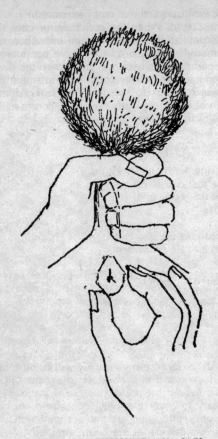

34. EXPRESSING ANAL SACS

6. The secretion normally is yellowish brown in color, ranging in consistency from watery to pastelike. The presence of pus or blood indicates that an infection is present and a veterinarian should be consulted.
7. If the anal area is irritated from the dog's licking or biting, apply an antiseptic skin ointment to relieve the irritation.
8. Wash the hair around the anus if the foul odor persists.

If impacted anal sacs are not emptied promptly, they can become abscessed. When the condition reaches this stage, treatment by a veterinarian is required. Abscesses may rupture spontaneously; or if they have not already opened, surgery may be necessary to drain the sacs. Treatment after drainage usually consists of injecting the sacs with antibiotics; this may be repeated several times until improvement is noticed.

ANIMAL BITES

(See "Wounds, Open.")

ARTIFICIAL RESPIRATION

Anything that stops breathing or reduces the oxygen supply to the lungs, making breathing difficult, should be considered a life-threatening respiratory emergency.

When breathing stops, the tissues and cells are denied oxygen. When its oxygen supply is stopped, a dog can die within 3 to 5 minutes. Because time is so important, artificial respiration should be started as quickly as possible in a respiratory emergency. Artificial respiration is a procedure that induces the flow of air into and out of the lungs when natural breathing stops or is insufficient.

Causes of Respiratory Emergencies

1. Obstruction by the tongue or by material. The latter includes partial or complete blockage of the air passage by food, pieces of toys, bones, plastic, or other solid articles; by fluids such as mucus, blood, or inhaled vomitus; by certain poisons; by swellings which occur after burns or eating certain types of plants; by insect stings or other allergic reactions. Obstruction can also result from injury by a direct blow.
2. Circulatory collapse (shock).
3. Asphyxia caused by inhalation of smoke, carbon monoxide, or other toxic gases, or by being trapped

in enclosures which do not contain enough oxygen to support life. Asphyxia from carbon monoxide and some other gases is heightened by a danger of explosion, for example, of combustible gases in mines and sewers, or the escape of natural or synthetically produced cooking gas in an enclosed area. The air in wells, sewers, mines, and old refrigerators and freezers may be depleted of oxygen. Without ventilation, a trapped animal will die quickly of asphyxia.

4. Poisoning by drugs that affect respiration. (See "Poisoning.")
5. External strangulation: hanging or being trapped by a collar that has caught on a fence or tree.
6. Severe chest injuries. (See "Chest Injuries.")
7. Drowning. (See "Drowning.")
8. Heart disease.
9. Electrical emergencies.

Symptoms of Respiratory Emergencies

- Breathing may be shallow or labored. The dog may struggle for breath with its mouth open.
- Breathing may stop.
- A bluish color to the tongue and inside the mouth and eyelids.
- Enlargement of the eye pupils (severe symptom).
- Loss of consciousness (severe symptom).

How to Give Artificial Respiration to a Dog

1. Remove or loosen the collar or anything tight around the dog's neck.
2. Lay the dog on its side on a firm surface. Extend the head and neck to help improve the airway to the lungs—*unless* there is a neck or back injury.
3. Open the mouth and pull the tongue forward. To help hold the tongue, use a gauze dressing, clean cloth, or handkerchief. (If there is a neck or back injury, open the mouth carefully, without moving the head.)
4. Use your fingers (wrapped in gauze or a handkerchief if possible) to quickly wipe off any mucus or foreign material inside the mouth.

56

5. **Place the palms of both hands on the chest behind the shoulder blades and in front of the last rib (Illus. 35) and:**

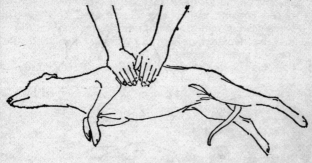

35. ARTIFICIAL RESPIRATION

   a. Press down *firmly* for 2 to 3 seconds.
   b. Release the pressure suddenly for 2 to 3 seconds.
   c. Repeat pressing and releasing every 5 to 6 seconds.
Remember: each movement should be vigorous. You want to press down sharply to compress the chest and empty the lungs of air, then release suddenly to expand the chest and fill the lungs with air.
6. If the chest has been injured (fracture, crushing injury, open wound), you must use another method to give artificial respiration, the mouth-to-nose technique:
   a. Pull the dog's tongue forward and to the side and close the mouth as well as you can.
   b. Cup your hands in an airtight circle and place them over the dog's muzzle (Illus. 36(a)) or take a deep breath and form an airtight seal with your mouth over the dog's nose (Illus. 36(b)).
   c. Blow into the dog's nostrils for 2 to 3 seconds.
   d. Remove your mouth for 2 to 3 seconds to permit air to be expelled from the dog's lungs.
   e. Repeat this procedure continuously. The amount of air you blow into the nostrils depends on the dog's size. Gentle puffs may be adequate for

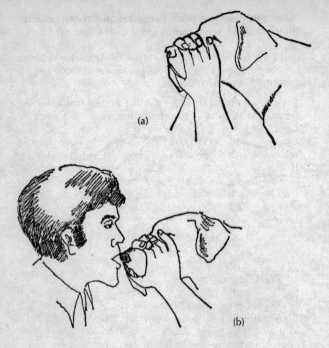

(a)

(b)

36. CUPPED-HANDS PROCEDURE

small dogs, but you may have to blow as hard as you can for large or giant breeds.

7. Continue either procedure until natural breathing resumes or a veterinarian pronounces the dog dead. Don't give up; it sometimes takes an hour or more to revive a dog.

8. If you get tired, have someone substitute for you.

9. Heart failure usually follows respiratory failure and often artificial respiration must be combined with external heart massage. (If you cannot detect a pulse or feel the heartbeat through the chest wall, see "Cardiac Arrest.")

10. When the dog revives, keep it warm and quiet.

11. Treat for shock if necessary. (See "Shock.")

12. Seek veterinary help as soon as possible. If necessary,

continue giving artificial respiration on the way to the hospital.

Caution: While performing artificial respiration, look and listen for air leaving the lungs. If you do not get an air exchange, try the following:

1. Reposition the head and neck for better airway to the lungs. *Do not move the head, however, if a neck or back injury is suspected.*
2. Check inside the mouth to see if you have missed removing any accumulated mucus or foreign materials.
3. If a foreign substance is causing obstruction of the airway, grasp the tongue and insert your index and middle finger into the dog's mouth. Slide your fingers around in the mouth as deeply as possible to try to remove the object.
4. If the object is a deep obstruction, as a last resort, place the dog on its side. Position the palms of your hands on the dog's body in back of the last rib. Press vigorously inward and forward. Release quickly, then press inward and forward again several times to force the lower chest to increase air pressure inside and dislodge the object (Illus. 42). *Do not perform this Heimlich maneuver, however, if there are severe chest, abdominal, or back injuries.*

AUTOMOBILE ACCIDENTS

What to Do If Your Dog Is Struck by a Moving Vehicle

Moving vehicles, especially cars, are responsible for more dog accidents and deaths than is any other kind of emergency. If your dog is struck by a car, the damage can be extensive. Correct first aid can help to save your dog's life.

1. The first thing to remember is that the dog is frightened and in pain. Use extreme caution when approaching it, because it may be confused and not know if you caused the accident or will inflict addi-

tional pain. *Every move you make must help comfort and reassure the dog.*

2. A dog that is frightened and in pain may try to bite. If necessary, apply a safety muzzle before you evaluate the extent of the injuries. (See "Handling and Restraint.")

3. Do not move the dog unless it is absolutely necessary. However, if the dog is in the middle of a street or highway, you must move it to safety. Grab hold of the loose skin at the back of the neck with one hand, and the skin over the back with your other hand. Pull the body evenly and gently onto a blanket, coat, jacket, or something similar that can be used to slide the dog out of the way of traffic. If you have nothing to use as a slide, gently and evenly pull the dog, keeping its body in a straight line, to safety.

4. Remove the collar or anything tight around the neck that obstructs breathing. If breathing stops, give artificial respiration. (See "Artificial Respiration.")

5. If there is profuse bleeding, control it immediately with an improvised pressure bandage. (See "Bleeding.")

6. A dog that is seriously injured or that has lost a great deal of blood will go into shock quickly. Check for signs of shock and do everything possible to help prevent or postpone its onset. Keep the dog quiet and cover it with a blanket, your jacket, or a coat to keep the body warm. (See "Shock.")

7. Next, check to see if any of the following are present:
   a. Spinal injuries.
   b. Head injuries.
   c. Chest injuries with crushing of chest.
   d. Abdominal injuries.
   e. Eye injuries (severe).
   Each of these (which can be looked up in the Contents) is a serious emergency and requires immediate treatment. There may be broken legs and other external injuries which will require treatment but are not life-threatening. *Remember: Saving your dog's life should be your first concern.*

8. Try to determine the extent of damage, and report it to your veterinarian immediately so that he or she can be adequately prepared for your arrival. *Do not*

60

leave your dog alone, for in its confused and dazed state, it may try to run away. If necessary, ask a bystander to call the veterinarian for you.

9. Do not give anything by mouth, as this can aggravate internal injuries.

10. Move the dog with extreme caution. (See "Emergency Transportation of Injured Dogs.") Proceed to the veterinarian at once. If you are away from home and do not know a veterinarian, phone the police and ask directions to the nearest veterinary hospital.

BLEEDING

In cases of severe injury where there is extensive and rapid loss of blood, *immediate action is necessary to prevent the dog from bleeding to death.* Regardless of what other injuries are present, stop or control massive bleeding first, treat for shock, and get to a veterinarian at once.

Symptoms

First aiders should be able to recognize different types of bleeding. *Bleeding from an artery:* Bright red blood spurts or gushes from the wound, synchronized with the heartbeats. Arterial bleeding is the most difficult to control. *Bleeding from a vein:* Darker red blood seeps in a steady flow from the wound. *Bleeding from capillaries:* Blood oozes slowly and steadily from several places on the wound's exterior. This type of bleeding occurs after minor cuts, scratches, and abrasions.

Materials Required to Control Bleeding

Sterile gauze dressings (or substitute dressings)
Cotton
Bandage
Instant cold compress or ice
Adhesive tape
Materials for tourniquet: pencil, stick, or similar object

Emergency Action

1. Careful handling is important. Do not move the dog more than is necessary.
2. Make sure breathing is not obstructed.
3. If the dog tries to bite, carefully tie a soft safety muzzle around the mouth. (See "Handling and Restraint.") When you handle a seriously injured dog, restraint should be as gentle as possible and should be used only when necessary. Don't cause additional upset to a freightened dog by applying excessive restraint.
4. Stop the bleeding with a pressure bandage:
   a. Place a sterile gauze dressing, clean cloth, handkerchief, or sanitary napkin directly over the wound.
   b. Apply firm pressure with your fingers or palm of your hand over the wound (Illus. 37). Continue the pressure for several minutes, allowing the blood to collect on the dressing and clot.
5. Bleeding from most small wounds will stop within a few minutes. When this happens, clean the wound thoroughly (see "Wounds, Open"), then dress and bandage (see "Bandaging").
6. If the bleeding does not stop and keeps coming through the pad, leave the original dressing in place and add a second dressing over the first. *Do not remove the original dressing and disturb the clot formation.* Keep adding one dressing on top of another

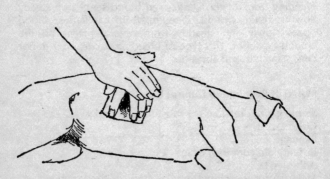

37. APPLYING PRESSURE BANDAGE TO STOP BLEEDING

until the bleeding is controlled. Continue direct pressure.

7. Bandage to keep the dressing in place.
8. Activate the instant cold pack or place some crushed ice in a plastic bag. Wrap either in a towel and apply immediately above the wound. This will cause a constriction of the blood vessels and help control the blood flow from the wound.
9. Unless you suspect a fracture, elevate the injured leg(s) higher than the heart. Gravity can help control the bleeding.
10. If the bleeding is still not controlled by direct pressure and elevation, apply pressure with your fingers at one of the body's pressure points (Illus. 38).

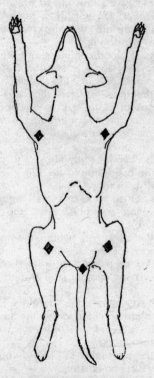

38. PRESSURE POINTS

a. To control bleeding in a front leg, press your fingers on the inside part of the leg just above the elbow on the brachial artery.

b. To control bleeding in a hind leg, press your fingers on the upper inside part of the leg on the femoral artery where it crosses the thigh bone.

c. To control bleeding of the tail, press your fingers on the coccygeal artery on the underside of the tail close to where it joins the body.

11. Use the pressure point technique in conjunction with direct pressure and elevation only to stop the bleeding. Release the pressure as soon as the bleeding stops.

12. Once the bleeding is under control, cover the wound with a sterile gauze dressing to prevent contamination. Remember: Do not lift or remove the original dressing and disturb the clot formation. Bandage firmly. (See "Bandaging.")

13. If rapid loss of blood continues and the dog's condition deteriorates, apply a tourniquet as a last resort. *Use a tourniquet only in a life-threatening emergency when all other methods have failed:*

a. Use strips of cloth, gauze, or bandage about 2 inches wide for the tourniquet band. If nothing else is available, use a soft nylon lead, a belt, or a piece of rope.

b. Place the band slightly above the wound.

c. Wrap the band around the dog's leg twice, then tie a half-knot (Illus. 39(a)).

d. Place a pencil, stick, or something similar on top of the loop and finish tying the knot on top (Illus. 39(b)).

e. Twist the stick and tighten the tourniquet just enough to stop the bleeding.

f. If the dog keeps moving its leg, keep the stick in place by tying another strip around the leg (Illus. 39(c)).

g. If the tissue below the tourniquet swells or becomes bluish in color, loosen the bandage slightly.

h. Apply instant cold pack or ice wrapped in a towel above the wound.

i. Leave the tourniquet in place if you can get to a veterinarian immediately.

j. If you cannot reach a veterinarian quickly, phone to report the condition and get instructions about loosening the tourniquet. To leave a tourniquet in place for long will stop the circulation to the injured area and cause extensive tissue damage.
14. Treat for shock if necessary. (See "Shock.")
15. Give first aid for other serious emergencies only.
16. Get the dog to a veterinarian immediately.

Internal Bleeding

Internal bleeding can result from a sharp blow or crushing injury from an automobile or other major accident. This is a serious emergency. When there is extensive blood loss, the dog will go into shock as its pressure falls. *Immediate treatment is necessary.*

Symptoms of Internal Bleeding

- White or pale gums.
- Rapid breathing.
- Coughing up red foamy blood.

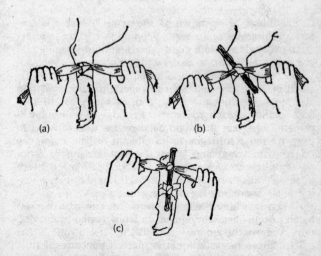

(a)   (b)

(c)

39. APPLYING TOURNIQUET TO STOP BLEEDING

- Weak pulse.
- Cold, clammy skin and extremities.
- Bleeding from nose, mouth, rectum.
- Blood in urine or bowel movements.

Emergency Action for Internal Bleeding

1. Remove the dog's collar or anything tight around the neck that might obstruct breathing.
2. Position the head to make breathing as easy as possible.
3. Cover the body with a blanket to keep the dog warm and quiet.
4. Do not give anything by mouth.
5. Treat for shock if necessary. (See "Shock.")
6. Get the dog to the veterinarian immediately. Move the dog carefully, preferably on a flat surface to avoid unnecessary shaking or abrupt movement. (See "Emergency Transportation of Injured Dogs.")

BLOAT

Canine bloat, also known as the acute gastric dilation-torsion syndrome is a puzzling condition which can affect deep-chested large and giant breeds without warning and can cause a torturous death within hours.

Bloat begins with an accumulation of gas in the stomach. The dog is unable to relieve the accumulation and the stomach begins to distend, causing great discomfort. As the stomach continues to enlarge, it pushes backward to press on the abdominal organs and forward to press on the diaphragm. In an attempt to gain relief, the dog tries to vomit and is unsuccessful. During the contractions to produce vomiting, the dog's stomach twists in some cases. If it does, the stomach is without an opening and cannot release its contents.

As the stomach swells (often to the size of a basketball), there is interconnected and progressive deterioration. The circulation of blood to the vital organs is impaired. Pressure on the diaphragm produces respiratory distress, with shallow, rapid breathing. The dog may go into shock from circulatory and respiratory failure. Eventually, due to lack of adequate blood supply to the vital organs—the kidneys, liver, and brain—shock and death ensue. Bloat is a life-threatening emergency which requires the immediate attention of a veterinarian.

Causes

The exact causes are unknown but some conditions thought to cause bloat are:

* Overeating.
* Abnormal swallowing of air.
* Trauma.
* Vomiting.
* Perverted or depraved appetite: eating feces, stones, bones, wood, and other foreign objects.
* Behavior disturbances.
* Vigorous exercise before or after eating.
* Excessive water drinking after eating or exercising.
* Hereditary predisposition.
* Abdominal surgery.

Symptoms (in Order of Progression)

1. The dog becomes uncomfortable and restless. It may pace about.
2. This is followed by excessive salivation or drooling.
3. Increasing dilation causes the abdomen to swell, especially just in back of the rib cage on the dog's left side.
4. The dog gags and swallows repeatedly, attempting to vomit.
5. The abdomen becomes tense and there is evidence of great pain.
6. At this stage, the dog may get up and lie down repeatedly.
7. Increasing dilation causes the stomach to press on the diaphragm. In an effort to gain relief, the dog sits or stands continuously.
8. Breathing becomes shallow and rapid.
9. The abdomen becomes very distended and sounds like a drum when tapped with your fingers.

10. The eyes have a staring look and the gums, inside of the mouth, and tongue may be dark in color.
11. The dog collapses and goes into shock.

Emergency Action

1. *Remember, bloat is a life-threatening emergency.*
2. Treat for shock. (See "Shock.")
3. Get the dog to a veterinarian at once. If you cannot locate your regular veterinarian, go to the nearest one. Treatment will be more successful if the dog is still physically strong. Delay may cause death, as the pathological changes that result from bloat are over-whelming, interconnected, progressive, and eventually irreversible.
4. Watch for signs of respiratory failure or cardiac arrest en route. (See "Artificial Respiration" and "Cardiac Arrest.")
5. Do not attempt home treatment unless you are given instructions by a veterinarian. Prepackaged bloat kits, available from veterinarians, are almost essential for bloat-prone dogs. It is important that before a bloat kit is used, a veterinarian explain its contents and demonstrate how the supplies can be used in an emergency to relieve accumulated gas in gastric dilation or torsion.

Dogs Most Susceptible to Bloat

1. Dogs 2 years of age or older.
2. Males (twice as often as females).
3. Deep-chested large and giant pure breeds and mixed breeds. The following purebreds have been affected by bloat:

Afghan Hound	Dalmatian
Basset Hound	Doberman Pinscher
Bernese Mountain Dog	English Bulldog
Bloodhound	English Setter
Borzoi	German Shepherd
Bouvier des Flandres	German Shorthaired
Boxer	Pointer
Bull Mastiff	Golden Retriever
Collie	Gordon Setter

Great Dane   Otter Hound
Great Pyrenees   Pointer
Irish Setter   St. Bernard
Irish Wolfhound   Scottish Deerhound
Labrador Retriever   Standard Poodle
Mastiff   Vizsla
Newfoundland   Weimaraner
Old English Sheepdog

4. Dogs that eat large quantities of commercial rations as the major part of their diet. Dogs that eat one meal per day are more susceptible than those eating two or three meals per day.
5. Dogs that drink excessive quantities of water after eating or exercise.
6. Dogs that exercise strenuously.
7. Dogs related to other dogs that have bloated.

BLOODY STOOLS

Causes

Blood in a dog's stool can be caused by several conditions, some of which are quite serious.

- Foreign objects in rectum.
- Poisoning (certain types).
- Accidents.
- Anal gland impaction.
- Cuts
- Internal parasites (hookworms).

Action

Unless the cause can be instantly and correctly identified and treated (see symptoms and treatment for subjects listed above), consult your veterinarian as soon as possible.

BURNS AND SCALDS

Animal burns most often result from contact with direct heat, flames, hot liquids, chemical agents, or electrical currents. A burn is an injury caused by dry heat, such as flames, while a scald is caused by moist heat, for example, having boiling water, tea, or coffee, or hot fat spilled on the body. Symptoms and emergency action are the same for burns and scalds. (Emergency treatments for burns from corrosive chemicals (acids, strong alkalis), frostbite or freezing, and contact with electrical currents are listed under "Burns, Chemical," "Frostbite or Freezing," and "Electrical Shock.")

Symptoms

Burns and scalds result in tissue destruction; the degree of damage depends on the depth and location of the injury, and the percent of body surface involved. Traditionally burns are classified by depth of injury from first degree (the mildest) and second degree to third degree (the most severe) but for simplicity, we will divide them into supercial and deep burns.

A superficial burn damages only the outer layers of the skin and is usually reddish. It may produce slight swelling, mild lesions (small, fluid-filled sacs), and peeling of the skin. The hair may be singed but as a rule it will be securely fixed in place. The pain may range from moderate to sharp; but usually a superficial burn will heal quickly with little treatment and no scarring.

A deep burn penetrates through the skin and destroys deeper tissues. Because there is extensive nerve damage, a deep burn is often less painful to the dog than a superficial burn. The burned skin may appear charred or pearly-white. Usually the coat is lost, and any remaining hair patches can be pulled out easily.

A deep burn not only destroys hair and skin, but tendons, muscles, and even bones. Complete destruction of the skin layers leaves large exposed areas from which body fluids can escape. A dog with deep burns will go into shock quickly, which can cause loss of life in the absence of immediate medical treatment. The greatest hazard, both early and late, is infection. In deep burns, bacteria can not only invade the surface tissues but can be absorbed into the bloodstream and produce septicemia, which is responsible for the greatest number of fatalities in burned dogs that survive the initial burn injury and shock period.

Prognosis

Burn outcome is more predictable than most other major injury outcomes. Some significant guidelines:

1. Age of the victim. Young adult dogs (with no pre-existing disease) respond more favorably to treatment than do very young or old dogs.
2. Percentage of body surface affected. When 15% or less of the body is involved, the burn usually can be treated successfully. When 15% to 50% of the body surface is involved, serious complications can result and even with proper medical treatment, the outlook for recovery is only fair. Deep burns involving more than 50% of the body, are usually fatal. Since the dog's pain and suffering will be intense, the owner should be compassionate and consider having the dog quietly put to sleep.
3. Pulmonary or respiratory complications from smoke inhalation.
4. Development of "burn shock." In severe burn cases, shock can be fatal.
5. Development of infection.

Materials Required for Superficial Burns

Instant cold compress or ice
Antiseptic skin ointment
Sterile gauze dressings
Bandage

Action for Superficial Burns

1. Muzzle the dog if necessary. (See "Handling and Restraint.")
2. Clip the hair from the burn and surrounding areas.

71

3. Gently wash the area with germicidal soap and water to prevent contamination.
4. If the burn is recent, help cool the area:
   a. Apply an instant cold compress wrapped in a towel; or
   b. Apply a clean towel or cloth that has been soaked in ice water and wrung out; or
   c. Immerse the burned area in cold (not ice) water. Cold therapy should be started within 10 minutes after the burn occurs, if possible.
5. Gently blot the area dry with sterile gauze dressings. Do not dry with cotton.
6. Apply a small amount of antiseptic skin ointment to the burn. Do not use grease, butter, margarine, lard, salad oil, or other home remedies: these can trap the heat, cause complications, and delay healing.
7. Cover lesions with dry sterile gauze dressings. Bandage to keep the dressings in place.
8. Consult your veterinarian for additional instructions.
9. Change dressings every 2 days. Check for infection. Before applying a new dressing, gently wash the affected area with germicidal soap and cool water, rinse well, and blot dry with sterile gauze.
10. If minor lesions are present, they usually dry to a thin parchmentlike crust in 3 to 5 days. Do not remove this crust: during the next few weeks it will separate naturally as the tissue is regenerated.

Materials Required for Deep Burns

Instant cold compress or ice
Sterile gauze dressings or substitute dressings
Clean towels or sheet
Blanket

Emergency Action for Deep Burns

1. If rescue from a fire has taken place, check the dog carefully for signs of smoke inhalation. (See "Poisoning: Inhaled; Poisons.")
2. Establish a clear airway and give artificial respiration if necessary. (See "Artificial Respiration.")
3. As soon as possible, cool the burned area to help

decrease the amount of heat in the deeper tissues:
  a. Activate instant cold compress, wrap in a towel, and apply over the injured area; or
  b. Soak towels in ice water, wring out excess moisture, and apply lightly to the burned area; or
  c. Submerge the burned area in cold (not ice) water. *Do not submerge the dog in cold water if more than 50% of the body is burned, as this can increase the tendency to shock. Instead, use (a) or (b).*
4. Do not apply antiseptic sprays or ointments, burn preparations, butter, lard, or other home remedies; they may interfere with the veterinarian's treatment.
5. Before you move the dog, cover the cold compresses or wet dressings with clean towels, sheets, or bandage to prevent contamination. Do not put pressure on the burned area.
6. Cover with a blanket to keep the dog warm. Watch for signs of shock and treat immediately if necessary. (See "Shock.")
7. Get the dog to the veterinarian immediately. Handle the dog gently and carefully when moving it to your car. (See "Emergency Transportation of Injured Dog.")

If a veterinarian cannot be reached within one hour, complete steps 1 through 6 and:
7. Keep the dog quiet and in a comfortable position. Keep the blanket wrapped around the body to prevent chilling. Provide gentle reassurance as the dog will be in great pain.
8. Check breathing frequently. If the dog stops breathing, start artificial respiration. (See "Artificial Respiration.")
9. Keep checking for signs of shock.
10. Do not give sedatives or other medication unless advised by your veterinarian.
11. If the dog is conscious and not vomiting, allow it to sip a salt and soda solution. The mixture recommended for burn patients by the American National Red Cross is 1 level teaspoon of salt and 1/2 level teaspoon of baking soda in a quart of cool water. Give 2 to 4 ounces every hour, depending on the dog's size, at home or on the way to the veterinarian. If vomiting occurs, discontinue the fluids.

12. Make every effort to get to a veterinarian as quickly as you can.

BURNS, CHEMICAL

Chemical burns occur when a dog comes into contact with chemicals containing strong acids or alkalis, both of which are caustic and fast-acting. Contact often occurs in garages or basements where chemicals are stored.

Symptoms

- Local pain.
- Reddened skin.
- Unusual odor of dog.
- Tissue damage—especially if the chemical has been on the skin for a long time.

Emergency Action

1. Muzzle or restrain the dog if necessary. (See "Handling and Restraint.")
2. Flush the skin, using a shower spray or hose, using plenty of cool water.
3. If the eyes are involved, flush with cool water under low pressure, holding the lids apart, *Rinse* for at least 5 minutes. Eye contact with chemicals requires the immediate attention of a veterinarian or veterinary ophthalmologist. (See "Eye Emergencies.")
4. Check the chemical's package or label and follow emergency instructions given for treating burns.
5. If there are no label instructions and the burning substance contained an alkali, after flushing the skin with water, rinse or sponge with a mixture of equal parts water and vinegar. *Do not apply this mixture before flushing the skin with water or you may aggravate the burn. Do not get the mixture into the dog's eyes.*
6. If the burning substance contained an acid, after flushing the skin with water, mix 2 to 3 tablespoons of baking soda per quart of warm water and rinse or sponge on the dog's skin.

7. After flushing the chemical off the skin, treat as directed for superficial or deep burns.
8. Treat for shock if necessary. (See "Shock.")
9. Get the dog to a veterinarian immediately.

CARDIAC ARREST

Cardiac arrest means that the heart has abruptly stopped beating. If you cannot feel the pulse over the femoral artery at the inside of the thigh on the back leg or detect a heartbeat on the left side of the lower chest wall just behind the elbow (see "Determining Your Dog's Heartbeat and Pulse" in Section II), the dog may be in cardiac arrest. *Act quickly.* External heart massage should be started as soon as you suspect cardiac arrest, for irreversible brain damage will begin after 3 to 4 minutes without oxygen.

Symptoms

- Shallow breathing.
- Absence of pulse in the femoral artery.
- Absence of heartbeat through the chest wall.
- Coldness of the skin.
- Respiratory arrest.
- Cessation of bleeding from wound, if any.
- Extreme dilation of pupils of the eyes.
- Loss of consciousness.

Emergency Action: External Heart Massage

1. Ensure an adequate airway. Remove the collar or anything tight around the neck that might obstruct breathing.
2. Place the dog on its right side on a firm surface.
3. The method of giving external heart massage varies with the size of the dog:
    a. For medium or large breeds: Make a fist and hit the chest once or twice in the area just behind the elbow. Then place the palm of each hand on the dog's chest, in back of the elbow (Illus. 40).

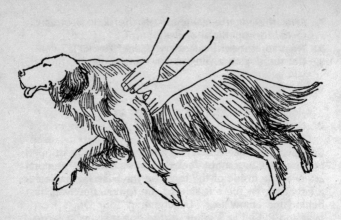

40. EXTERNAL HEART MASSAGE OF LARGE AND MEDIUM-SIZED DOG

Apply pressure on the heart by pushing downward; then completely release the pressure of your hands.

b. For small breeds: Make a fist and hit the chest once or twice in the area just behind the elbow. Then place the palm of one hand on each side of the chest (Illus. 41). Apply pressure on the heart by pushing downward with the hand on top and using the hand under the chest to support the dog's body; then completely release the pressure of the top hand.

4. Repeat either procedure every 1 to 2 seconds about 15 times.

5. Breathing also stops in cardiac arrest cases. If no help is available, stop external massage after 15 compres-

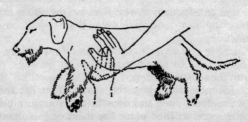

41. EXTERNAL HEART MASSAGE OF SMALL DOG

sions to give artificial respiration for 2 to 3 breaths. (See "Artificial Respiration.")

6. Resume external heart massage for another 15 compressions. Stop again for 2 to 3 breaths of artificial respiration.

7. If help is available, combine artificial respiration with external heart massage at the rate of 4 to 5 compressions to 1 breath.

8. During external massage, try to detect a pulse or feel the heartbeat in the chest wall. Any pulsation—even a slight flutter—is a sign to continue.

9. Continue external massage until the heart resumes beating or until you have determined unmistakably that, after a reasonable amount of time, the heart has stopped beating.

10. Get the dog to a veterinarian as quickly as possible. Continue external massage en route if necessary.

Caution: External heart massage should be given only when the dog's heart has stopped beating. Do not give it in any emergency if there is an easily detectable heartbeat.

CHEST INJURIES

Emergencies of the chest include open or penetrating wounds and crushing injuries; each of these requires treatment as quickly as possible. The lungs may be constricted by fluids, blood, or air which has leaked into the chest cavity through an opening in the lung's exterior. A constricted lung causes serious breathing difficulties and is a serious emergency that requires immediate medical attention.

Open and Penetrating Chest Wounds

These can be caused by major accidents, wounds from gunshots and other sharp objects or instruments, and other forms of violence. Open and penetrating wounds are life-threatening emergencies: once the chest wall is opened, air can flow into the cavity around the lungs during inhalation and cause the lungs to collapse. Deep wounds may cause damage to the heart, lungs, or blood vessels resulting in violent bleeding.

Symptoms of Open and Penetrating Chest Wounds

- Deep open wound.
- Sharp object penetrating chest.
- Breathing difficulties.
- Breathing may sound like a sucking noise through the chest wall.
- Collapse
- Shock.

Materials Required for Open and Penetrating Chest Wounds

Dressings and bandage as necessary for wounds
Large nonporous covering for an open wound, such as a sheet, cloth, piece of aluminum foil, plastic, or as a last resort, paper
Blanket

Emergency Action for Open and Penetrating Chest Wounds

1. Maintain a clear airway. Breathing must not be obstructed.
2. Do not apply a safety muzzle.
3. Open wounds: For a deep open area, the first thing you must do is to close the wound to prevent air from entering the chest cavity:
   a. Place a large nonporous covering (a clean sheet or other cloth, piece of aluminum foil, plastic, or as a last resort, piece of paper) over the opening, making an airtight closing.
   b. Cover the pad with bandage or tape to hold it in place. The seal should not permit the entry of air, but do not bandage so tightly that breathing is obstructed.
   c. If necessary, use the palm of your hand to close the wound until you can locate bandage.
   d. Place the injured side down if possible.

78

4. Penetrating wounds: If an object or instrument is still intact, do not disturb it—otherwise, you may cause additional damage and violent bleeding. Apply dressings, packing, and bandage to hold the object in place. Do not move the dog unless absolutely necessary.
5. Treat for shock if necessary. (See "Shock.")
6. Handle and move the dog as carefully as possible. (See "Emergency Transportation of Injured Dogs.")
7. Get the dog to a veterinarian immediately. Phone the hospital in advance, if possible, so that treatment can be given as soon as you arrive.

Crushing Chest Injuries

Crushing chest injuries can be caused by automobile or major accidents, falls from heights, severe blows or kicks, or other forms of direct violence. These injuries are painful and make breathing difficult. Usually this type of injury includes rib fractures, which increase the amount of pain and make breathing even more difficult.

Symptoms of Crushing Chest Injuries

- The dog may stand or sit with forelegs or all four legs held wide apart, head extended, and mouth open.
- Attempts to breathe are made with abdominal muscles.

Materials Required for Crushing Chest Injuries

Dressings and bandages as required for injuries
Blanket (for shock, if necessary)

Emergency Action for Crushing Chest Injuries

1. Keep the air passages clear. Elevate the head to make breathing as unobstructed as possible.
2. Do not muzzle the dog.
3. Carefully dress and bandage any wounds. Apply bandage carefully so that breathing is not obstructed.
4. If the injury is on both sides, place the dog in the most comfortable position. If the injury is on one side, if possible have the dog lie with the wound side down.

5. Keep the dog warm and quiet. Watch for signs of shock. (See "Shock.")
6. Get the dog to a veterinarian as soon as possible. Move with extreme care. (See "Emergency Transportation of Injured Dogs.")

CHOKING

(See also "Foreign Objects, Swallowed or Embedded.")

Choking occurs when food or a foreign object obstructs the esophagus and prevents the dog from breathing. Quick action is important: a few minutes of lack of oxygen can cause the death of a choking dog.

Symptoms

- Profuse salivation.
- Gulping and gasping for breath.
- Gagging and attempts at vomiting.
- Anxious attitude—pawing at the throat and mouth.
- Inside of the mouth and tongue may turn blue.
- Collapse.
- Loss of consciousness.

Materials Required for Emergency Action

Forceps or long-nosed pliers
Sterile gauze dressing or handkerchief

Emergency Action; The Heimlich Maneuver

There are several ways to deal with choking:

1. Open the mouth. If necessary, keep a grip on the dog's tongue with a gauze or handkerchief. Reach inside and remove the obstruction with forceps, long-nosed pliers, or your fingers.
2. If the obstruction cannot be removed from the air passage, the Heimlich maneuver, a technique developed for dislodging food or foreign obstructions in human throats, can be applied to dogs (or cats):

a. Rest the dog on its side on a firm surface (table-top for small breeds, floor for larger dogs).
b. With one of your hands on top of the other (Illus. 42(a)), place the heel of your bottom hand into the midline of the abdomen, below the rib cage (Illus. 42(b)).
c. *Press vigorously into the abdomen with a quick upward thrust. Release; then press into the abdomen once again with a quick upward thrust.* Repeat several times if necessary. The purpose of this maneuver is to exert pressure that forces the abdomen upward, compresses the air in the lungs, and expels the object caught in the breathing passage.
d. As you perform the Heimlich maneuver, have an assistant open the dog's mouth, grasp its tongue and lower jaw (hold with a gauze dressing if necessary), and probe the area with fingers to locate and remove the object.

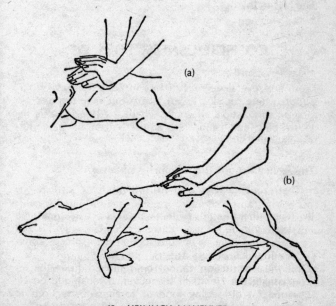

42. HEIMLICH MANEUVER

e. If breathing has stopped, after the object is dislodged and removed give artificial respiration until normal breathing resumes. (See "Artificial Respiration.")
3. The dog should see a veterinarian as soon as relief is obtained, as performing the maneuver can result in injury to the dog. *However, the dog will survive only if its airway is quickly cleared!*

COMA

(See "Consciousness, Loss of.")

CONCUSSION

(See "Head Injuries.")

CONSCIOUSNESS, LOSS OF

There are several degrees of loss of consciousness, from stupor, where the dog is not awake but may respond to forceful stimulation, to coma, where the dog appears to be sleeping and cannot be aroused even by powerful stimulation.

Causes

Loss of consciousness may be the result of primary or secondary causes. *Primary causes* include injuries and diseases which immediately affect the dog's nervous system, such as:

- Concussion, fractured skull, or other head injuries.
- Brain diseases (hemorrhage, tumor, abscess, meningitis, encephalitis).
- Seizures.
- Certain types of poisoning.

Secondary causes include injuries and diseases which first affect other systems of the body before attacking the nervous system, such as:

- Shock.
- Suffocation.
- Electrical shock.
- Heatstroke.
- Exposure to extreme cold.
- Liver or kidney disease.
- Heart or circulatory failure.
- Metabolic problems (low blood sugar, diabetes, low calcium).
- Severe dehydration.

Investigation*

Special physical signs are liable to occur in unconscious dogs and these should be noted during examination:

1. Respiration: This may be shallow or deep, rapid or slow.
2. Pupils: The pupils normally become smaller when exposed to light. It should be noted whether the pupils are large or small and whether they are equal in size. Their reaction to light should be tested.
3. Corneal reflex: Attempts to touch the cornea normally result in blinking. This reflex should be tested, but care must be taken not to injure the delicate cornea.
4. Depth of unconsciousness: In stupor, the animal can be roused with difficulty, the pupils respond to light, and the corneal reflex is present. In coma, the animal is more deeply unconscious and cannot be roused, the pupils are dilated, and the corneal reflex is absent.
5. Pulse: The rate and character should be determined.
6. Odor of breath: In cases of poisoning, the odor may give a clue as to the cause, and characteristic odors may be noticed in cases of uremia and diabetes.

* R. D. Pinniger, ed., *Jones's Animal Nursing*, © 1976 British Small Animal Veterinary Association. Pergamon Press, fully rev. 2d ed., 1976.

7. Convulsions: Violent, irregular, involuntary movement of the limbs.
8. Paralysis: Loss of use of muscles.
9. Incontinence: Involuntary passing of urine or feces.
10. Rigidity: Involuntary spasm of muscles, so that they appear stiff and firm and cannot be relaxed.

Emergency Action

1. Remove the dog's collar or anything tight around the neck that might obstruct breathing.
2. If there are no severe head, neck, or spine injuries, position the head to make breathing as easy as possible. Open the mouth, clean out all foreign matter, and pull the tongue forward.
3. Treat for shock. (See "Shock.")
4. Do not give anything by mouth.
5. Check for head, spine, or other serious injuries before moving the dog. If any of these are present, move the body carefully on a firm surface. (See "Emergency Transportation of Injured Dogs.")
6. Get the dog to a veterinarian immediately, as this is a serious emergency.

CONSTIPATION

Constipation is the collection of hard fecal matter in the colon which may stem from a variety of causes. The condition is characterized by painful, difficult, and irregular passage of stools.

Causes

- Insufficient bulk in the diet.
- Eating quantities of foreign material (bones, hair, wood, etc.) which compact in the intestines.
- Lack of exercise.
- Overfeeding (especially older pets or dogs that receive little exercise).

Constipation can also occur when the passage of stool is hindered by:

1. Enlarged prostate gland.
2. Tumors of the rectum or colon.
3. Anal gland abscesses.
4. Pelvic fractures.
5. Perineal hernia.
6. Temporary paralysis (from car accidents, back injuries, etc.).
7. Nerve damage (loss of nerve supply to the colon decreases the capability of normal passage of stools).
8. Megacolon (excessive dilation of the colon).

Symptoms

- Severe straining.
- Abnormally dry or hard stool.
- General listlessness.
- Bleeding from the rectum (not always present).

Action and Prevention

1. Your veterinarian may recommend a change in diet or suggest that you add more water to the dog's present diet to make it moister. Foods like liver and milk soften the bowels and may be added to the regular diet several times a week.
2. Do not give bones that can be eaten. Bones are wonderful to help prevent boredom but they should be chewed, not eaten by a dog!
3. Give the dog a *mild* laxative or lubricant such as Milk of Magnesia or mineral oil. Mineral oil is given by adding it to the dog's food (about 1 to 2 teaspoonsful per 10 pounds of body weight). It should not be given separately, for it can cause pneumonia if inhaled. It's important to know that mineral oil should be given sparingly, because it interferes with the absorption of fat-soluble vitamins.
4. Your veterinarian may prescribe a medication that will help soften the stool or a bulk producer which will mix with intestinal fluids to produce a soft stool. This encourages bowel movement.
5. Assuming the dog is in good health, begin a program of regular exercise. Interesting walks, mild exercise periods in the backyard, playing with safe toys, and

the like will contribute to your dog's good mental and physical well-being.

6. If constipation is acute, use an infant suppository or give an enema. (See "How to Give an Enema" in section II.) The enema may be repeated once; if relief is not obtained after the second enema, consult your veterinarian.

Other conditions can cause a dog to strain and appear to be trying to make a bowel movement. Before assuming that the dog is constipated, the pet owner should be aware that straining can be caused by bladder infection or other urinary disease, by an intestinal inflamation, or by outside impaction of the hair around the anus.

On long-haired breeds with an abundance of coat around the anal area, the hair can become tangled or clogged with remains from a previous bowel movement which has hardened into a mass; then the tangled hair or hardened mass seals the anal opening so securely that a bowel movement becomes impossible. When this happens, the dog will strain and cry out, often licking or biting the area in an attempt to gain relief. If this is not attended to immediately, it can develop into a painful condition. Trim away the tangled hair with a blunt-tipped scissors or clippers, or soak the hardened mass in warm water until it softens and can be removed. It may be necessary to shampoo and dry the hair around the anal area afterward. Apply an antiseptic skin ointment if the anal area is inflamed from the dog's licking or biting. Periodically scissor or clip the hair around the anus to keep the outward impaction from recurring.

CONVULSIONS

A convulsion is a short, violent attack of unconsciousness accompanied by stiffening of the body and followed by jerking, uncontrollable movements and frothing of the mouth. Most convulsions last a few seconds to a minute or so, then subside. Usually the seizure has stopped by the time you are able to reach a veterinarian by phone. A mild convulsion seldom causes death but should be reported to your veterinarian. He or she will make an appointment to examine the dog in the near future, to try to establish the cause of the seizure and possibly to begin treatment. If, however, a convulsion lasts for more than 5 minutes or if the dog has repeated seizures, it should be considered an emergency which requires immediate attention by a veterinarian.

Causes

- Trauma.
- Head injuries from major blows or accidents.
- Epilepsy.
- Hereditary predisposition.
- Brain damage from a previous viral or bacterial disease, such as canine distemper.
- Tumors.
- Low blood sugar.
- Low calcium (sometimes occurs after whelping a litter of puppies).
- Liver or urinary disease.
- Exposure to certain drugs, such as amphetamines.
- Exposure to certain poisons, such as lead, strychnine, ethylene glycol, insecticides containing organophosphates, chlorinated hydrocarbons, Warfarin or other anticoagulant rodenticides, metaldehyde.

Symptoms

Seizures may be preceded by:

- Dazed expression.
- Licking of the lips.
- Light muscle twitching.
- Restlessness and nervousness.
- Salivation.
- Personality changes.

During the seizure, the dog may experience:

- Violent muscle spasms.
- Jerking, uncontrollable movements.
- Overwrought activity.
- Jaws opening and closing rapidly.
- Profuse drooling; a frothing at the mouth.

- Falling to the floor.
- Stiffness of legs.
- Loss of urinary or bowel control.
- Rolling eyes.
- Loss of consciousness.

Seizures may be followed by:

- Confusion.
- Dazed expression.
- Wobbly movement.
- Hiding.
- Hunger.
- Drowsiness.

Materials Required for Emergency Action

Blanket

Emergency Action

1. Maintain a clear airway. Loosen the collar or anything tight around the dog's neck that might obstruct breathing.
2. Cover with a blanket or towel to keep the dog warm and quiet.
3. Do not restrain. Above all, do not muzzle the dog.
4. Prevent the dog from injuring itself or an onlooker. Inside the house, keep the dog away from stairs or other potential hazards.
5. Try not to touch the dog's face. Do not put medication or liquids into the mouth.
6. Keep children away.
7. After the seizure subsides, keep the dog warm and quiet and allow it to rest.
8. Check breathing closely. If necessary, give artificial respiration. (See "Artificial Respiration.")
9. If the convulsion lasts for more than 5 minutes or if the dog has repeated seizures, see a veterinarian immediately.
10. Every seizure, no matter how mild, should be reported to your veterinarian. If the dog is to be examined in the near future, do some homework and provide your veterinarian with a complete history of

seizures (symptoms, frequency, duration); changes in eating, drinking, or sleeping habits; personality changes; changes in urination or bowel movements; records of vaccinations; previous illnesses and injuries; and, if possible, whether there is a history of seizures in the dog's family.

Seizures can be controlled by medication, but it may take time to find the correct drug or combination of drugs that will be effective for your dog. Don't be discouraged. Give plenty of love and understanding to your dog while a therapeutic regimen is being established.

COUGHING

A cough may be temporary and trivial, but more often it is a symptom of many illnesses, including:

1. Roundworm infestation.
2. Heartworm infestation.
3. Infectious tracheobronchitis (often called "kennel cough").
4. Tonsillitis.
5. Laryngitis.
6. Pharyngitis.
7. Asthma.
8. Lung ailments (pleurisy, pneumonia).
9. Canine distemper.
10. Obstruction in the throat.
11. Heart trouble (especially in older dogs).

Because of the diversity of these illnesses, it is important to identify the characteristics (moist, dry, hacking, etc.) of the cough. If the cough persists, the dog can become so worn out that other symptoms may be noticed. Consult your veterinarian immediately, for your dog may be suffering from a serious illness.

DEHYDRATION

Loss of body fluids from severe diarrhea, fever, heat-stroke, diabetes, distemper, starvation, wound drainage, excessive secretion of urine, and vomiting can cause dehydration, which occurs when a dog discharges more fluid than it takes in. The signs of dehydration are not noticeable until a considerable fluid loss (equal to about 5% of body weight) has occurred. If your dog is dehydrated, it may have been ill for some time and may require immediate medical attention.

Symptoms

- Changes in the skin: loss of elasticity. To determine dehydration, pinch a fold of skin on the dog's side near the middle of the back. It should go back into position immediately. If it is slow to go back or remains pinched together, the animal is dehydrated.
- Dryness of mouth tissue.
- Eyes appear sunken into skull.
- Shock or involuntary muscle twitching (not always present).

Emergency Action

1. Remove the dog to a veterinarian for fluid therapy at once.

DIARRHEA

Diarrhea is frequent evacuation of soft or watery stools. It can result from a variety of causes:

1. Change of food or water.
2. Overeating or overdrinking.
3. Eating contaminated foods or garbage.
4. Internal parasites (worms).
5. Intestinal irritations caused by bacterial or viral infections.

6. Psychological stress.
7. Food or drug allergies.
8. Systemic diseases (hepatitis, leptospirosis, uremia).
9. Certain types of poisons.
10. Liver disease.

In chronic diarrhea, the cause must be determined and treated. Usually diarrhea is not considered an emergency unless it occurs in young puppies or old, debilitated pets.

Symptoms

* Frequent, foul-smelling watery or bloody stools.
* Listlessness.
* Fever (not always present).
* Vomiting (not always present).

Materials Required for Management

Kaopectate®, Donnagel®, or Pepto-Bismol®
Antiseptic skin ointment

Management

1. Withhold all solid food for 12 to 24 hours to allow the stomach to rest.
2. Do not give milk. Allow the dog to drink water, but not in excessive quantities. If the dog wants to over-drink, allow it to lick ice cubes.
3. Administer an antidiarrhea preparation (Kaopectate®, Donnagel®, Pepto-Bismol®, or similar preparation), 1 to 2 teaspoonsful per 10 pounds of body weight every 4 to 6 hours.
4. After the fast, feed soft bland food such as cottage cheese, cooked egg, rice, boiled beef (drained of liquids), and farina. Large amounts of muscle meats, meat by-products, and coarse cereals should be avoided. Maintain the bland diet for 4 to 5 days. The following soft, bland low-fiber diet has been provided by Dr. Mark L. Morris, Jr.:

$^1/_2$ cup farina (Cream of Wheat®) cooked to
   make 2 cups
$1^1/_2$ cups creamed cottage cheese
1 large egg, hard-cooked
2 tablespoons brewer's yeast
3 tablespoons sugar
1 tablespoon corn oil
1 tablespoon potassium chloride
2 teaspoons dicalcium phosphate

Add a balanced vitamin-mineral supplement sufficient to provide the daily requirement for each vitamin and trace mineral. Cook farina according to package directions. Cool. Add remaining ingredients to farina and mix well. Yield: 2 pounds.

Feed a sufficient amount to maintain normal body weight.

Body Weight	Approximate Daily Feeding
(lbs.)	(lbs.)
5	$^2/_3$
10	1
20	$1^2/_3$
40	$2^3/_4$
60	$3^3/_4$
80	$4^3/_4$
100	$5^1/_2$

5. If the dog has a sore anal area from frequent diarrhea, apply antiseptic skin ointment to relieve the irritation.
6. If the diarrhea persists for more than 36 to 48 hours, consult your veterinarian. Diarrhea is often a simple functional disorder, but prolonged passage of loose stools may indicate the presence of some serious problem. If possible, take along a stool sample at the time of examination; it may help your veterinarian diagnose and treat the condition.

DROWNING

The general assumption that dogs are natural swimmers is not always true. Most dogs can swim well naturally; but until you learn your dog's capabilities in water, don't force it into a life-threatening situation. The danger of drowning is often present when a dog falls out of a pleasure boat or jumps or falls into a steep-sided pool. If water sports are an important part of your family's life, learn to take precautions to protect your dog from drowning.

Symptoms

- Since air in lungs has been replaced by water, breathing may be slight or labored or stop completely.
- The lips and tongue may turn a deep red or blue in color.
- The dog may be unconscious.

Materials Required for Emergency Action

Instant hot compress or hot-water bottle
Blankets

Emergency Action

1. Open air passages immediately. Lift the dog by its hind legs and hold it upside down for about 30 seconds to allow the water to drain out of the mouth and nose. If the dog is too heavy or too large to hold upside down, lay it on its side on a slanted surface with the head lower than the rest of the body to encourage drainage.
2. Make sure the tongue is pulled forward to facilitate breathing.
3. If breathing has stopped, start artificial respiration. (See "Artificial Respiration.")
4. Cover the dog with a blanket to help prevent pneumonia.
5. Activate instant hot compress or use hot-water bottle for additional warmth.

93

6. Consult your veterinarian immediately.
7. Even if regular breathing resumes and dog appears to be well, it should be examined for possible complications.

DRUG OVERDOSE

Dogs or puppies, out of curiosity, or boredom when left alone with nothing to interest them, often get hold of medication bottles. If the bottle is plastic, it's possible for the dog to chew through it and swallow the contents. Depending on the type and amount of medication swallowed, drug overdose can be a serious emergency. *Always keep medicines stored where your dog cannot reach them.*

Symptoms

These vary depending on the type and amount of drug swallowed but can include any of the following:

* Restlessness.
* Nausea.
* Confusion.
* Excessive thirst.
* Dizziness.
* Lack of coordination.
* Difficulty in swallowing or breathing.
* Trembling and chills.
* Slow pulse and respiration.
* Lowered temperature—cool skin and extremities, pale tongue and mouth tissues.
* Convulsions.
* Loss of consciousness.
* Coma.
* Shock.

Materials Required for Emergency Action

Emetic to induce vomiting (see "Poisoning")
Blanket

Emergency Action

1. If the dog is conscious, induce vomiting by giving an emetic. (See "Poisoning.")
2. For any drug overdose, call your local Poison Control Center *immediately* for the antidote.
3. Certain drugs paralyze brain centers which control respiration. If breathing has stopped, give artificial respiration. (See "Artificial Respiration.")
4. Treat for shock. (See "Shock.") Keep the dog warm by wrapping it with a blanket.
5. Get the dog to a veterinarian as soon as possible.

EAR EMERGENCIES

Ear emergencies usually involve injuries to the earflaps, which have a tendency to bleed profusely. They can be the result of bites by another animal, cuts, tears from barbed-wire fences or other sharp objects, foreign bodies (thorns, etc.), or self-inflicted severe scratching.

Symptoms (Depending on Injury)

- Swelling and/or redness of earflap tissue.
- Crying out when the ear is touched.
- Excessive scratching or rubbing of the ear.
- Shaking the head. (Persistent shaking, rubbing, or scratching can cause the blood vessels of the earflap to rupture, fill with blood, and swell to a tumorlike mass called a hematoma.)
- Bleeding (limited or profuse).

Materials Required for Ear Injuries

Sterile gauze dressings
Bandage
Germicidal soap

Emergency Action for Ear Injuries

1. If the injury is a minor cut with limited bleeding,

treat as instructed in "Wounds, Open: Minor Wounds."

2. If bleeding is profuse, use sterile gauze dressings and apply direct pressure over the injured area. For severe tears and profuse bleeding, consult a veterinarian immediately, as sutures will be necessary.

3. When the bleeding stops, remember that the injury can be aggravated by the dog's natural tendency to shake its head, so you will have to steady the injured ear with a firm bandage.

4. Place a sterile gauze pad on top of the dog's head. Lay the injured earflap back onto this.

5. Place another sterile gauze pad on top.

6. Wrap bandage around the head, leaving the other ear free to help keep the bandage in place and prevent it from sliding backward. Be sure the bandage is not tight enough to restrict breathing. Steps 4, 5, and 6 are shown in Illus. 24.

7. Apply adhesive tape to keep the bandage in place.

8. Consult your veterinarian for additional medical treatment, if necessary. A hematoma requires treatment by a veterinarian.

ELECTRICAL SHOCK

Electrical shock most often occurs when a dog (especially a teething puppy) chews through a live wire.

Caution: Do not touch dog while it is in contact with electrical current.

Symptoms

- Weakness
- Paleness of lips, mouth, and eyelid tissues.
- Moderately cool skin and extremities.
- Low body temperature.
- Collapse.
- Loss of consciousness.
- Burns inside the mouth.

Materials Required for Emergency Action

Pencil, stick, broom handle, or other nonconductor of
  electricity
Towel and blanket

Emergency Action

1. If the wire is still inside the mouth or touching the
   body in any way, don't handle the dog until the cord
   is disconnected from its power source.
2. If you can reach the plug, pull it out or remove the
   fuse if you know instantly which one controls that
   particular electrical current; *but, don't waste time
   hunting for the fuse box when the dog's life is at
   stake!*
3. If you cannot locate the fuse box or unplug the cord
   from its electrical outlet, wrap a heavy terry towel
   around your hand or use a pencil, stick, broom handle, or other nonconductor of electricity to push the
   wire out of the dog's mouth or to move the body
   away from the frayed cord.
4. Keep the dog warm. Wrap the body with a blanket
   for additional warmth.
5. Treat for shock if necessary. (See "Shock.")
6. If breathing stops, administer artificial respiration. (See
   "Artificial Respiration.")
7. If the heart stops beating, give external heart massage.
   (See "Cardiac Arrest.")
8. When breathing resumes, check inside the dog's
   mouth for burns. They are not of first importance but
   will need treatment later.
9. Consult veterinarian immediately.

EYE EMERGENCIES

Eye Injuries Which Require Emergency Action

1. Foreign bodies in the eye.
2. Scratches, lacerations, or penetrating wounds of the
   cornea.
3. Chemical burns and irritation.

4. Lacerated or bleeding eyelids.
5. Bruises and/or bleeding from severe blows.
6. Prolapsed eyeball (eyeball out of its socket).

If your dog experiences any of these, immediate emergency action can help to prevent permanent damage. (For eye problems which are not considered emergencies, see "Applying Topical Medications: Medicating the Eyes" in section II and "Grooming: The Eyes" in section IV.)

Any dog can experience an eye injury, but the short-nosed breeds such as the Bulldog, Pekingese, Shih Tzu, Pug, Brussels Griffon, and Boston Terrier, with large round eyes set in shallow sockets, seem to be more susceptible to damage.

Foreign bodies in the eye cause pain and irritation and produce excessive tearing, blinking, and rubbing; there is an added danger that the object will become embedded in or scratch the cornea or conjunctiva. Allowing a dog to ride with its head out the window of a car is a common cause for foreign bodies being blown into the eye. Don't allow it.

Eye injuries cause a great deal of pain and discomfort. The dog may paw or scratch at its eyes to gain relief, and in doing so, cause additional damage, permanent scarring, and conceivably a partial loss of vision. An effective way to prevent further injury until treatment is obtained is to bandage and/or tape the dog's front and back feet; this may also be necessary after treatment, to discourage scratching during the healing process. (For other suggestions for preventing self-mutilation, see "Bandaging.")

Because the eye is a fragile and sensitive organ, examination and emergency treatment should be performed as carefully as possible.

Symptoms (Depending on Injury)

- Blinking and sensitivity to light.
- Profuse tearing of one or both eyes.
- Red or irritated eyeball.
- Torn or bleeding eyelid.
- Pawing or scratching at eyes or head.
- Bloodshot parts of the eyes that normally are white.

- Swelling around the eyes.
- Third eyelid prolapsed.
- Pupils very small.
- Eyeball out of its socket.

Foreign Bodies in the Eye

Foreign bodies such as dust, grit, wood splinters, grass or other seeds, thorns, hair, and flakes of paint or metal can be blown or rubbed into the dog's eyes.

Materials Required for Foreign Bodies in the Eye

Q-Tips, gauze dressings, clean handkerchief or tissue
Warm water or commercial rinsing solution such as Dacriose or Dissol (rinsing solution should be used warm or at room temperature)

Emergency Action for Foreign Bodies in the Eye

1. If the dog resists and you cannot examine the eye, apply a safety muzzle; wrap a towel or blanket around the body to keep the dog from struggling or have an assistant restrain the head. (See "Handling and Restraint.")
2. Examine the eye under a bright light by gently opening the eyelid.
3. Flush the eye with warm water or a commercial rinsing solution, allowing the liquid to drain down and away from the eye. The water or rinsing solution can be applied by an eyedropper or rubber bulb syringe, or by wetting cotton balls and letting the liquid drop into the eye.
4. If you can locate the foreign body (which is often behind the third lid), gently lift it out of the eye with a moistened Q-Tip, corner of a gauze dressing, or clean handkerchief or tissue. *Do not rub over the eye and do not use dry material to remove the object.*
5. If the foreign body seems to be embedded, keep the eye cleansed and open and consult a veterinarian as soon as possible.

Scratches, Lacerations, or Penetrating Corneal Wounds

These are painful and serious emergencies which can result in partial loss of vision. They must be treated immediately by a veterinarian.

Materials Required for Scratches, etc.

Warm water

Emergency Action for Scratches, etc.

1. Flush the dog's eyes with lukewarm water applied by an eyedropper or by saturating cotton and allowing the water to drop into the eye.
2. If a penetrating object is still in the eye, do not remove it.
3. Keep the eye uncovered. Many first-aid guides recommend covering the eye with a moistened gauze dressing, but this will probably do more harm than good.
4. Get the dog to a veterinarian immediately.

Chemical Burns and Irritations

A dog's eyes can be burned or irritated by contact with soaps, shampoos, insecticides, or other chemical irritants. Immediate treatment is necessary, as some chemical irritants can cause extensive damage to the cornea or conjunctiva.

Materials Required for Chemical Burns and Irritations

Warm water

Emergency Action for Chemical Burns and Irritations

1. Flush the eye(s) with warm tap water under low pressure, holding the lids apart. Water may also be applied by an eyedropper or by saturating cotton and allowing the water to drop into the eye. Whatever method is used, flushing should begin immediately after irritation and continue for at least 5 full minutes. Do not allow the contaminated flushing solution to run into the other eye if only one eye is affected.
2. Get the dog to a veterinarian immediately.

Lacerated or Bleeding Eyelids

Lacerated and bleeding eyelids can result from the bites of cats or other animals, from serious accidents, and from cuts from hooks or wire. These injuries cause all kinds of tearing, and sutures may be necessary.

Materials Required for Lacerated or Bleeding Eyelids

Instant cold compress or ice
Q-Tips or gauze dressings

Emergency Action for Lacerated or Bleeding Eyelids

1. Bleeding will usually stop with cold applications. Activate instant cold compress, wrap in a towel, and apply over the lid for a few minutes. Use crushed ice if cold compress is not available.
2. Cleanse the wound with warm water. Apply the water by soaking cotton and letting it drop onto the injured area.
3. Use a Q-Tip or corner of a gauze dressing to remove any debris from the wound.
4. Get the dog to a veterinarian immediately.

Bruises and/or Bleeding from Severe Blows

Serious injuries from direct blows to the head or eye, accidents, and other severe injuries may produce bruising above and below the eyes or may rupture the blood vessels of the eyeball and produce hemorrhage. These injuries should receive immediate veterinary attention; the eye's structure may be torn or dislocated.

Materials Required for Bruises/Bleeding

Instant cold compress or ice

Emergency Action for Bruises/Bleeding

1. Activate instant cold compress or place some crushed ice in a plastic bag. Wrap either in a towel and place over the injured area as soon as possible to arrest swelling and bleeding. If neither cold compress nor

ice is available, wet a sanitary napkin with cold water and place over the injured eye.
2. Get the dog to a veterinarian immediately.

Prolapsed Eyeball

A dog with large eyes set in shallow sockets, Pekingese, Pug, Shih Tzu, Bulldog, etc., may have an eyeball thrust out of its socket by severe blows from automobile accidents or fights with other dogs. This emergency requires immediate treatment by a veterinarian. There is an added danger because the eyeball begins to swell as soon as it pops out of its socket. The greater the swelling, the more difficult the eyeball is to replace; surgery may be required.

Materials Required for Prolapsed Eyeball

Gauze dressings, clean cloth or handkerchief
Maple syrup, saturated sugar solution or water-soluble jelly (such as K-Y jelly)

To make a saturated solution, place some sugar in a bowl and add just enough water to make a syrupy consistency.

Emergency Action for Prolapsed Eyeball

1. Dampen a gauze dressing or clean cloth or handkerchief with maple syrup, saturated sugar solution, or water-soluble jelly. Place the dressing over the prolapsed eyeball to prevent further contamination and maintain moistness on the way to the veterinarian.
2. Assure an adequate airway. Make sure breathing is unobstructed.
3. Treat for shock if necessary. (See "Shock.")
4. Go to a veterinarian immediately.

If You Cannot Reach a Veterinarian Quickly

1. Keep the surface of the eyeball moistened with maple syrup, saturated sugar solution, or water-soluble jelly.
2. Open the eyelids as far as you can and with gentle

pressure use a moistened Q-Tip or gauze dressing, trying to replace the eyeball in its socket if possible.
3. Close the lid and apply a gauze dressing coated with saturated sugar solution over the eye.
4. Maintain an adequate airway.
5. Treat for shock. (See "Shock.")
6. Get the dog to a veterinarian as quickly as possible.

FACE AND NECK EMERGENCIES

Injuries from automobile and other accidents, falls from high places, and kicks or other severe blows may cause extensive damage to the face and neck, including broken jaw, deep cuts, lacerations and abrasions, and nosebleeds. These injuries can be serious, and the dangers are even greater when profuse bleeding and swelling are present, as the air passage may become blocked, which can be especially hazardous for the short-nosed breeds such as the Pekingese, Shih Tzu, and Bulldogs, in which any difficulties around the throat can cause added respiratory stress. A nosebleed can also be caused by an abscess, a tumor, or a foreign object caught inside the nostril.

Symptoms of Face and Neck Emergencies

- Difficulty in breathing.
- Bleeding.
- Blood from nostrils.
- Jaw hanging open.

Materials Required for Emergency Action for Nosebleed

Sterile gauze dressings
Bandage or handkerchief, scarf, napkin, etc.
Instant cold compress or ice

Emergency Action for Nosebleed

1. Keep the dog quiet. Place in a sitting position with the head forward.
2. Apply direct pressure by pressing bleeding nostrils together with your thumb and index finger.

3. If one nostril is bleeding, pack it with sterile gauze. Leave the packing in place for 1 to 2 hours. Do not pack both nostrils.
4. Activate instant cold compress or place ice in a plastic bag. Wrap either in a towel and place around the top and sides of the dog's nose.
5. Keep the dog's head bent slightly forward to prevent blood from seeping into the throat.
6. If the bleeding does not stop, consult your veterinarian as soon as possible.

Emergency Action for Other Face and Neck Injuries

(See also: Head Injuries.)

1. Keep air passages clear. Open the mouth, pull the tongue forward, and clean out all foreign substances. Remove the collar and carefully position the head so that breathing is unobstructed. (Do not move the head if a neck fracture is suspected.)
2. If breathing stops, give artificial respiration. (If the jaw is fractured, it may be difficult to do this. See "Artificial Respiration.")
3. If the injuries are serious, especially from an automobile accident, severe blow, or fall, treat for shock if necessary. (See "Shock.")
4. Apply pressure bandages to control bleeding when necessary. Do not allow bleeding to interfere with breathing. Turn or position the head, *unless a neck fracture is suspected,* to allow blood or saliva to drain out instead of draining into the throat.
5. If the lower jaw is fractured and hanging open:
   a. Use a length of gauze bandage or fold a handkerchief, napkin, or scarf into a cravat-shaped bandage.
   b. Place the middle part of the bandage beneath the lower jaw.
   c. Bring the ends to the top of the muzzle and tie them together *loosely*. The purpose is not to close the mouth completely but only to give support and prevent further damage.
6. Deep neck wounds may involve major arteries and veins and may be difficult to control. Exert firm pres-

sure over the wound and do not remove the pressure until you reach a veterinarian. Do not apply a circular bandage around the dog's neck.
7. Get the dog to a veterinarian immediately. Move the dog with extreme care.

FOOT INJURIES: CUTS, PUNCTURES, OR OBJECTS IMBEDDED IN FEET OR PADS

Broken glass, wood slivers, tacks, nails, thorns, grass seeds, cinders, and other road debris are some of the foreign objects that can cause injury between a dog's feet or pads.

Symptoms

- Limping.
- Licking or chewing the foot.
- Affected area becomes swollen and hot.
- Pus discharge (not always present).
- Bleeding (deep cuts).

Materials Required for Emergency Action

Sterile gauze dressings
Bandage
Adhesive tape
Germicidal soap
Antiseptic for wounds
Scissors
Q-Tips, forceps, tweezers, or needle

Emergency Action for Deep Cuts

1. If the bleeding is profuse, stop it as soon as possible. (See "Bleeding.")
2. Perform emergency action as at "Wounds, Open."
3. Severe cuts usually will need to be sutured. Consult your veterinarian as soon as possible.

Emergency Action for Punctures

1. A foot puncture is a small opening made when a pointed object or instrument pierces or perforates the paw or pad. Although the wound opening is small, the performation can cause internal bleeding and/or infection.
2. Small puncture wounds are sometimes difficult to locate. If the dog is a hairy breed, remove some of the coat with clippers or scissors to locate the puncture.
3. Perform emergency action as at "Wounds, Open: Minor Wounds."

Emergency Action for Objects Embedded in or Between Feet or Pads

Foreign objects that become embedded in or between a dog's foot or pads cause irritation and infection. They should be removed as soon as possible:

1. Restrain the dog if necessary. (See "Handling and Restraint.")
2. Small embedded objects can be difficult to locate between the toes or pads. If the dog is a hairy breed, remove some of the hair with scissors or clippers to make it easier to find and remove the foreign object. Afterward, wash the area carefully with germicidal soap and water. Rinse and dry thoroughly.
3. Examine the affected area carefully under a good light. If you can see the foreign object, remove it with a Q-Tip or sterilized forceps, tweezers, or needle. (Wash the instrument, then soak in alcohol for sterilization.) A large foreign object that is deeply embedded, such as a piece of broken glass or nail, may seriously damage internal tissues and should be removed by a veterinarian. However, before moving the dog to the veterinary hospital, pack the foot with gauze bandage to hold the object steady and protect tissues from further damage.
4. Examine the area carefully to be sure that all traces of the object have been removed. Apply an antiseptic. If necessary, bandage the foot to prevent contamina-

tion and to keep the dog from licking the area during healing. (See "Bandaging.")

5. The wound should be cleaned, dried, medicated, and bandaged frequently as it heals. Watch for signs of infection. (See "Wounds, Open: Infected Wounds.") Consult a veterinarian if infection persists.

FOREIGN OBJECTS, SWALLOWED OR EMBEDDED

Some of the more common foreign objects swallowed by dogs are bones, toys or parts of toys, children's playthings, buttons, stones, nails, pins, needles, plastic objects, pencils, erasers, bottle caps, and stockings, as well as large pieces of food. The number of items in and around the house that a dog can chew and swallow is uncountable. If you own a young puppy aged 3 to 6 months that is teething (puppy teeth being replaced by adult teeth) and likely to chew to relieve the misery of gum irritation, or a young adult dog that spends much time alone and chews out of curiosity or boredom, read the suggestions in "Toys During the Teething Process" and "Providing Safe Toys," both under "Care of the Mouth" in section IV.

Slivers of wood or glass, thorns, fishhooks, porcupine quills, and other items may become embedded in the skin. Larger objects such as nails, scissor blades, knives, arrows, and pieces of metal can become deeply embedded through accidents.

Symptoms of Foreign Objects in Mouth or Throat

* Rubbing head on the ground.
* Pawing or scratching at the mouth.
* Excessive salivation.
* Coughing.
* Gasping or gulping for breath.
* Bluish color to inside of mouth and tongue.
* Choking (a serious emergency).

Symptoms of Foreign Objects in Stomach or Intestines

- Abdominal discomfort.
- Excessive vomiting (sometimes bloody).
- Blood from rectum or in bowel movement.
- Object visible under and through skin.
- Shock.

Materials Required for Foreign Objects in the Mouth

Gauze dressing or handkerchief
Tweezers, forceps, or long-nosed pliers

Emergency Action for Foreign Objects in the Mouth

1. If the dog is fussy, wrap its body in a towel or blanket for restraint. (See "Handling and Restraint.")
2. Open the mouth as far as possible and examine the teeth, gums, tongue, roof of the mouth, under the tongue, and back of the throat under a bright light. If the dog is uncooperative, hold the tongue with a gauze dressing or clean handkerchief to keep it from slipping.
3. Remove any foreign objects with your fingers, tweezers, forceps, or long-nosed pliers.
4. If the object is lodged deep in the throat and the dog is choking, *fast action is necessary*. (See "Choking.")

Emergency Action for Swallowed Objects

1. Do not give anything by mouth (including a laxative) unless advised by a veterinarian.
2. If the object is small and not sharp, watch the dog's bowel movements to see if it has passed through the digestive tract. If the object is not discharged within two days, consult a veterinarian.
3. If the object is sharp (such as a pin or needle), *take the dog to a veterinarian as soon as possible*.
4. If the dog has swallowed a string or thread, this can be serious. As the string passes through the digestive tract, contractions around it can draw the intestines into accordionlike pleats. The string can also cut the intestinal wall.

a. If the string is hanging out of the rectum, cut off the excess. Do *not* pull it out.
b. If part of the string is hooked around a tooth or the tongue and the rest has been swallowed, cut the string. Do *not* pull it out.
c. Observe the bowel movements to determine if the string passes out. If it does not come out within 24 hours, consult your veterinarian.
5. Treat for shock if necessary. (See "Shock.")

Materials Required for Foreign Objects Embedded in the Skin

Liquid antiseptic for flushing

Emergency Action for Foreign Objects Embedded in the Skin

1. If the object is close to the skin surface, remove it with your fingers, tweezers, or forceps.
2. Treat as instructed at "Wounds, Open."
3. If the object is a fishhook:
   a. Flush first with liquid antiseptic.
   b. Push the barb through the skin until the point appears.
   c. Cutoff the hook with pliers or wire clippers.
   d. Flush with antiseptic a second time.
   e. Push the shank back through the original opening and remove it.
   f. Clean the wound with germicidal soap and water. Apply antiseptic.
   g. This is a painful process and may have to be done under anesthesia by a veterinarian. Always consult a veterinarian: this type of wound often becomes infected because the fishhook is contaminated. Antibiotic treatment may be necessary.
4. For porcupine quills, see "Porcupine Quills."

Materials Required for Impaled Foreign Objects

Sterile gauze dressings
Bandage

Emergency Action for Impaled Foreign Objects

1. *Do not attempt to pull out the object.* To do so may cause additional damage and hemorrhage.
2. Muzzle and restrain the dog if necessary. (See "Handling and Restraint.")
3. If the object is long and slim, try to cut or snap it apart with pliers or your fingers. (Remember, however, to leave the object projecting 1 or 2 inches above the wound.)
4. Pad sterile gauze dressings around the object to keep it in place.
5. Bandage to secure dressings around the object. Apply bandage carefully, so that it does not put pressure on the object and force it inward.
6. Treat for shock if necessary. (See "Shock.")
7. Get to a veterinarian immediately. Move the dog as carefully as possible.

FOUL ODORS

(See also "Skunk Odor.")

Dogs sometimes roll in fertilizer, feces, or other offensive substances. While this is not a medical emergency, the pet owner will want to take quick action to remove the unpleasant "after-smell," especially if the dog is usually allowed on the sofa, bed, or other furniture.

An effective way to neutralize offensive odors is to shampoo the dog (twice, if necessary) and rinse well. Towel-dry the hair. Mix about 5 ounces of Massengill douche powder or liquid (available at most pharmacies) into 1 gallon of warm water. Pour or sponge the mixture over the dog, taking care not to get it into the eyes. Do not rinse. Allow the mixture to dry naturally on the hair. After the dog is dry, brush its hair.

It may be necessary to repeat the procedure.

FRACTURES, DISLOCATIONS, SPRAINS, AND STRAINS

Fractures

A fracture is a crack or break in a bone. Most fractures are caused violently: by automobile or other severe accidents, sharp blows or kicks, and injuries resulting from jumping or falling.

Broken legs seem to occur most often. It may be difficult to determine if a leg is broken; diagnosis may have to be confirmed by X ray. If you see a dog's leg hanging limply, unable to support its weight, a fracture should be suspected and a veterinarian consulted as soon as possible.

There are three types of fractures:

1. Simple fracture: The bone has one complete break and does not pierce the skin. However, there will be tissue damage in the area of the break.
2. Compound fracture: The bone has a complete break and protrudes through the skin. As a result of the bone being exposed, the skin and muscles may be torn or punctured, and bacteria may enter the tissues and cause infection.
3. Comminuted fracture: The bone is broken in several places. This type of fracture may be simple or compound.

Symptoms of Fractures

- Intense pain and swelling in the affected area.
- Limping.
- Loss of function: leg hanging and unable to support dog's weight.
- Bone protruding from skin in some instances.
- Sound of bones grating together.
- Apparent differences in length, shape, and angulation of corresponding bone on opposite leg.

Materials Required for Broken Leg

Sterile gauze dressings

Bandage or strips of cloth to use as ties
Material for padding: bandage underwrap, cotton batting
Adhesive tape
Splints (see below)

Emergency Action for Broken Leg

If a fractured skull, neck, or back is suspected, see "Head Injuries," "Face and Neck Emergencies," or "Spinal Injuries." The dog must be moved on a solid surface to keep the body and head from bending or twisting.

1. Maintain an adequate airway. Remove the collar or anything tight around the neck that might obstruct breathing.
2. The dog will be in great pain and may try to bite. If necessary, apply loose gauze safety muzzle. (See "Handling and Restraint.")
3. Place the dog in a comfortable position on its side with the broken leg on top.
4. If the dog is lying on a street or highway, immediately move it to safety. Grab hold of the loose skin at the back of the neck with one hand and the skin over the back with your other hand. Pull the body evenly and gently onto a blanket, coat, jacket, towel, or something similar that can be used to slide the dog out of the way of traffic. If you have nothing to use as a slide, gently and evenly pull the dog, keeping its body in a straight line, to safety.
5. Give first aid for profuse bleeding, shock, or other emergencies.
6. Keep the dog quiet. Do not turn, twist, or move the broken leg.
7. *Do not attempt to reset the break.* This should be done under anesthesia by a veterinarian. If a bone is exposed, control the bleeding, then cover the torn or punctured area with large sterile gauze dressings and bandage to help prevent further infection.
8. Apply a temporary well-padded splint to immobilize the leg to prevent additional damage until you can reach a veterinarian. Fractures of the lower leg should be supported by a splint. Fractures of the upper leg, close to where it joins the body, are difficult to recognize and/or immobilize. These should not be

splinted but the dog must be handled with great care and moved on a temporary stretcher if possible. (See "Emergency Transportation of Injured Dogs.")

9. When it is necessary to restrict the movement of an injured leg, you will have to improvise a splint from anything close at hand, such as pieces of board, a ruler, straight sticks, heavy cardboard cut into strips, corrugated cardboard carton bent to form a three-sided box, tongue depressors, yardstick broken into pieces, or rolled-up towels, newspapers, or a magazine.

   a. Ideally, the splint should be long enough to immobilize the joint above and below the fracture on each side of the leg.

   b. The area between the splint and the dog's skin should be well padded with bandage underwrap, cotton batting, gauze, cloth, tissues, paper towels, etc.

   c. If you are using rigid objects, you will need two separate splints, one on top of the leg and the other underneath. Splints made from towels should be folded into a horseshoe shape and then placed around the injured leg (Illus. 43). Newspapers or a magazine should be rolled around the injured leg (Illus. 44).

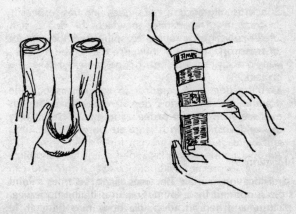

43. TOWEL SPLINT   44. NEWSPAPER SPLINT

d. Wrap bandage around the splint (tape the beginning and end of the bandage) or tie the splint to the leg at several points above and below the break. If possible, do not apply bandage, tie, or tape over the area of the fracture, for fear of causing complications. Apply sterile dressing, if available. Illus. 45 shows the leg splinted and tied.

e. Be sure the bandage or ties are not applied so tightly that circulation stops. Check for tissue discoloration or excessive swelling. If these symptoms appear, loosen the tie or bandage and reapply.

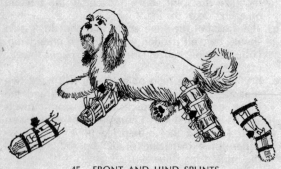

45. FRONT AND HIND SPLINTS

10. Shock usually accompanies body injuries, especially in fractures. The manner in which the dog is handled—splinting or failure to splint and the method of transportation—will influence the degree of shock. Act quickly to prevent or postpone shock. (See "Shock.")

11. Get the dog to a veterinarian as soon as possible. Handle and move the dog carefully, avoiding unnecessary movement of the injured part. (See "Emergency Transportation of Injured Dogs.")

Dislocations

In a dislocation, a bone becomes displaced from a joint. It's often difficult for a lay person to distinguish between a fracture and a dislocation; diagnosis may have to be confirmed by X ray. Dislocations can occur as a result of:

1. Violence: Automobile accidents, sharp blows or kicks, jumping or falling from considerable heights.
2. Recurring dislocations caused by the progressive degeneration of the joint capsule.
3. Genetic deformities.

In the dog, the most common dislocations occur in the hip, shoulder, elbow, or stifle joint. In any dislocation, the dog should be handled with great care to prevent tearing of the surrounding tissue and ligaments and additional damage to the nerves and blood vessels in the area.

Symptoms of Dislocations

- Swelling.
- Pain.
- Limping.
- Tenderness when affected joint is touched.
- Apparent differences in length or shape of corresponding area on the opposite side of the body.
- Bulging or distorted joint.
- Dog holding leg off the ground (kneecap dislocation).

Materials Required for Dislocations

Cold compresses or ice
Splints as necessary

Emergency Action for Dislocations

1. Do not attempt to reposition the dislocation at home. This will cause additional injury and great pain.
2. If the limbs are involved, follow emergency treatment for fractures.
3. If the shoulder or hip joint is involved, move the dog carefully to avoid additional injury.
4. Apply cold compresses or ice packs to help relieve pain.
5. Consult your veterinarian immediately. While it is not a life-threatening emergency, any dislocation should be examined by a veterinarian as soon as possible. Treatment is based on repositioning the dislocation; this will have to be done with the dog anesthetized. If treatment can be given within 24 hours of the injury, the dislocation can often be corrected without

surgery. However, if the bone is difficult to reposition or if it has a tendency to dislocate again, surgery will be necessary for permanent correction.

Sprains

A sprain is an injury to a joint ligament. There usually is a partial tearing and stretching of the supporting structures and blood vessels as well as damage to the soft tissues around the joint. Sprains can be caused by overexercise, twisting a limb beyond its normal range of motion, violent blows or kicks, or sudden twisting, jumping, or falling. In the dog, areas most likely to be affected are the shoulder, pastern (on the front leg), and stifle and hock joints (on the back leg). Because it may be difficult to determine if the injury is a simple fracture, dislocation, or sprain, X-ray examination may be necessary.

Symptoms of Sprains
- Swelling (developing shortly after the injury occurs), caused by damaged structures around affected joint.
- Tenderness and pain when affected joint is moved or touched.
- Limping.

Materials Required for Sprains

Instant cold compress or ice
Instant hot compress or warm moist compresses
Towel
Splints as necessary

Emergency Action for Sprains

1. Restrict movement as much as possible if a leg is affected.
2. If necessary, apply a splint to rest the leg.
3. Activate instant cold compress or place crushed ice in a plastic bag. Wrap the cold pack or ice bag in a towel and place it over the sprain for 15 to 20 minutes every 2 to 3 hours to reduce the swelling. This should be done over a period of 24 hours.
4. Depending on the severity of the sprain, after 24 hours you can follow with warm compresses.

5. Consult a veterinarian if the sprained area continues to be painful and swollen.

Strains

A strain is a muscle-tendon injury. Strains are caused by unexpected movements, resulting in a wrench which may be violent enough to stretch or tear the muscle or muscle-tendon unit. Strains can result from overexertion, especially in racing or hunting dogs, when the muscles are in poor condition or not sufficiently warmed up before an event.

Symptoms of Strains

- Lameness.
- Tenderness and pain when affected area is moved or touched.
- Slight swelling.

Materials Required for Strains

Instant hot pack or warm moist compresses
Splints as necessary

Emergency Action for Strains

1. Restrict movement as much as possible if a leg muscle is involved.
2. If necessary, apply a splint to rest the leg.
3. Activate instant hot compress and wrap in a towel, or place warm moist towels around the injury for about 15 to 20 minutes every 2 to 3 hours. Continue the warm applications until pain and discomfort are alleviated.
4. Consult a veterinarian if pain and lameness persist after a few days.

There is a long-established standard for suspected fractures, dislocations, and sprains: "If there is any uncertainty, splint the victim before moving." Even if a wrong decision is made and a splint is not necessary, it will not harm the victim.

FROSTBITE, OR FREEZING

Frostbite or freezing is an injury to the tissues which occurs when a dog is overexposed to cold. Usually the extremities—the toes, foot pads, tip of tail, tips of the ears—are affected first. The amount of damage depends on how long the animal is overexposed. Severe frostbite or freezing can occur when animals have been injured outdoors in cold weather or caught in wildlife traps or in other circumstances that prevent normal circulation.

Symptoms

- Cold, pale skin.
- After warming, the skin may be sensitive, red, and scaly. It may swell and then dehydrate and wrinkle.
- Severe frostbite may cause the skin to loosen and scale off.

Materials Required for Emergency Action

Instant hot compress, heating pad, or hot-water bottle
Towels
Blanket
Vaseline® or bland ointment
Thermometer

Emergency Action

Move the dog to a warm place and take immediate steps to rewarm it. Handle the dog gently, as frostbite can cause a great deal of pain.

1. If the frostbite is mild, use an instant hot compress, hot-water bottle, or heating pad. Warm the affected parts slowly and steadily; don't try to thaw them too quickly.
2. Do not cause friction by rubbing or massaging the frostbitten parts in an attempt to increase circulation.
3. After warming, cover the affected areas with a thin layer of Vaseline® or other bland ointment to prevent additional damage.
4. If the frostbite is severe, take the dog to a veterinarian

as soon as possible. Don't attempt further emergency treatment at home unless you cannot get professional help in a hurry. Protect the affected areas from injury during handling and transportation.

5. If a veterinarian cannot be reached, rewarm the frozen parts as soon as possible by immersing the dog in warm water. Afterward, dry gently with towels and warm air from a blow dryer if you have one.

6. Do not rub or massage the thawed parts. After drying, wrap the dog in a blanket to keep it warm.

7. An animal suffering from severe frostbite has low body temperature and can go into shock quickly. If this happens, begin emergency treatment for shock. (See "Shock.")

8. If breathing has stopped, start artificial respiration. (See "Artificial Respiration.")

9. Consult a veterinarian as soon as possible. He or she may prescribe antibiotics to help prevent infection and/or sedatives to reduce pain. There is a danger that the thawed parts will become red and swollen with accumulated fluids, or that the skin will peel off and leave exposed areas. It will take several days to determine if the tissue is healing properly. Unfortunately, if the tissue does not heal, gangrene may develop and amputation may be necessary. Keep the dog warm during recuperation, as continued exposure to cold will delay healing.

GENITAL ORGANS, INJURIES TO THE

Injuries to a dog's genital organs may be caused by tears from barbed-wire fences, severe blows, kicks, and lacerations, or other injuries by sharp instruments.

Symptoms
- Excruciating pain.
- Profuse bleeding.
- Swelling and redness of the area.

Materials Required for Emergency Action

Sterile gauze dressings
Instant cold compress or ice

Emergency Action

1. Muzzle or restrain the dog, if necessary. (See "Handling and Restraint.")
2. Control bleeding first. Cover the injury with a sterile gauze dressing and apply pressure with your hand. (See "Bleeding.")
3. Treat for shock if necessary. (See "Shock.")
4. Clean and dress minor wounds. (See "Wounds, Open: Minor Wounds.")
5. Activate instant cold compress or place a little crushed ice in a plastic bag. Wrap either in a towel and apply to injured area to help reduce swelling.
6. Consult your veterinarian as soon as possible.

HEAD INJURIES

(See also "Face and Neck Emergencies.")
Concussion, compression, skull fractures, hemorrhage, and other serious injuries to the skull and brain can be caused by severe blows, automobile accidents, falls from heights, etc. Open head wounds, including small ones, tend to bleed profusely. Deep wounds can be complicated by the presence of skull fragments or other foreign substances. *Head injuries are serious emergencies which require immediate treatment by a veterinarian.*

Symptoms (Depending on Part of Brain Affected)

- Slow, shallow breathing.
- Weakened pulse.
- Vomiting.
- Dilated pupils or pupils unequal in size.
- Involuntary rapid movement of the eye ball(s) (nystagmus).
- Bleeding or clear or blood-tinged fluid draining from nose, ears, or mouth.

- Paralysis of one side of the body.
- Loss of balance.
- Loss of bladder and bowel control.
- Loss of consciousness (partial or total).
- Coma.
- Shock.

Materials Required for Emergency Action

Sterile gauze dressings
Bandage
Board or other firm surface

Emergency Action

1. Place the dog on its side.
2. Keep air passage clear. Open the mouth and clear out all foreign substances and pull the tongue forward. Loosen the collar and carefully place the head so that breathing is unobstructed and accumulation of fluids in the mouth and nose is prevented.
3. If breathing stops, give artificial respiration. (See "Artificial Respiration.")
4. Watch for loss of consciousness. (See "Consciousness, Loss of.")
5. Keep the dog warm and quiet. Treat for shock. (See "Shock.")
6. For bleeding wounds:
   a. Place sterile gauze dressings over the wound and apply slight pressure to stop the bleeding. *The pressure should be gentle, to prevent further brain damage.*
   b. When the bleeding is controlled, do not clean the wound. Should the skull be fractured, doing this can cause brain contamination.
   c. Use bandage to keep the dressing in place and provide additional pressure. Do not bandage tightly.
7. If possible, move the dog on a board or other rigid surface to support the spinal column. (See "Emergency Transportation of Injured Dogs.")
8. Get the dog to a veterinarian immediately.

Note: Even if you suppose the wound is minor, consult

a veterinarian. A condition which may appear minor to a nonmedical person could develop into a life-threatening situation within 24 hours.

HEART STOPPING

(See "Cardiac Arrest.")

HEATSTROKE (HYPERTHERMIA)

Heatstroke occurs when a dog retains too much heat in its body. It is made more severe by lack of water.

Dogs maintain their body temperatures in a number of ways. When they become overheated, they disperse heat by panting and a certain amount of perspiration. However, dogs do not perspire through the pores of their skin like people. They release body heat less efficiently than man by perspiration only through their tongues and pads of their feet. A brief exposure to excessive heat may cause temporary panting and rapid breathing. A dog can cope with temporary high temperatures; for the more it pants, the more relief it gets. But exposure to high temperatures for a long time may result in heat prostration.

Causes

1. Confinement in poorly ventilated enclosures (a car parked in direct sunlight; a cramped traveling container) for too long.
2. Leaving the dog outdoors for a long time without adequate shade.
3. Excitement, overexercising, or working during hot weather.

Prevention

1. If you must travel with your pet in hot weather, provide adequate ventilation inside the car. Be prepared

for emergencies. Take along a supply of drinking water. Keep instant cold packs in the glove compartment for immediate use.

2. If you are traveling to a picnic, dog show, or other outing in hot weather, don't have the inside of the car too cold. When you arrive at your destination and the dog goes out into the heat, it can suffer too when subjected to such drastic changes in temperature.

3. Avoid strenuous exercise or walking your pet for long distances in direct sunlight. Do these activities in early morning or at sundown.

4. Don't take your pet along with you to outings and leave it in the car in hot weather unless you are sure you can park in a shaded area and safely leave the windows partly open. A car in direct sunlight gets hot inside very quickly—in a matter of minutes, interior temperatures can reach 110°F.

5. If you live in a year-round warm climate and often take your dog along in the car, consider purchasing reflective window covering to help lower the car's interior temperature without disturbing driving vision. This material can be purchased at any hardware store and cut to the size of your car windows in a few minutes.

Symptoms

- Elevated body temperature—often as high as 110°F.
- Rapid heart rate.
- Difficulty in breathing; panting or gasping for air.
- Wide, dilated eyes; a dazed expression.
- Staggering gait.
- Lying down or tendency to fall down easily.
- Convulsions or collapse.
- Pale or grayish mucous membranes.
- Vomiting (not always present).

Materials Required for Emergency Action

Thermometer
Cold compresses (2) or ice
Disposable enema

Emergency Action

Take immediate steps to reduce your dog's temperature to normal. Excessively high temperatures can be tolerated for only a short time before severe central nervous, heart, and brain damage will result.

1. Move the dog away from the heat to a cool or shady place, if possible.
2. Activate instant cold compresses. Place one compress on the back of the neck and the other on the dog's abdomen. If cold compresses are not available, use ice packs or soak the dog in cold water.
3. Take the temperature. (See "How to Take Your Dog's Temperature." in section II.)
4. Administer cool-water enema to help lower the internal temperature.
5. Be careful not to let the body temperature go too low, which might put the dog in shock. To avoid shock, after emergency procedures have been started, take the rectal temperature often to be sure it is lowering to within the normal range of 100.5°F to 102.5°F. Once the temperature lowers, check to see that it does not rise again suddenly or continue to drop.
6. Get the dog to a veterinarian immediately.

Dogs Most Susceptible to Heatstroke

- Dogs with short muzzles (Pekingese, Pug, Shih Tzu, Boxer, Bulldog, etc.).
- Overweight dogs.
- Dogs with heavy coats.
- Young puppies.
- Older pets.
- Pets with heart or kidney problems.

HIVES

(See "Allergy/Allergic Reactions.")

INSECT BITES AND STINGS

Symptoms of Common Insect Bites (Fleas, Lice, Mosquitoes, Flies, Gnats, etc.)

- Pain in affected area.
- Intense itching. The dog may bite and scratch its body, causing additional damage to the skin.

Materials Required for Common Insect Bites

Flea shampoo, powder, or spray (for fleas or lice)
Instant cold compress or ice
Calamine lotion

Action for Common Insect Bites

1. Fleas or lice: Remove insects by using a flea shampoo, powder, or spray. Follow manufacturer's instructions carefully.
2. Mosquitos, flies, gnats, and other common insects:
   a. If swelling is present, apply cold compress or ice to the affected area for about 10 minutes.
   b. Cover affected area with Calamine or other soothing lotion.

Facts About Common Insects

1. The adult flea is a dark brown, hard-skinned insect with a narrow body. It is wingless but has strong legs which enhance its ability to leap. A flea is capable of leaping about 14 inches horizontally and 7 inches vertically.
2. The flea bites by piercing the dog's skin and inserting its syringelike mouth. When it locates a blood vessel, it sucks the dog's blood. During feeding, flea saliva, which contains a chemical substance which causes itching, is introduced into the wound.
3. Some dogs become hypersensitive to flea saliva and develop a chronic condition called flea allergy dermatitis. The dog's fierce scratching and biting produces loss of hair and causes the skin to become thick, red, and infected, most often on the back just in

front of the tail, on the abdomen, or between the legs. The condition requires veterinary treatment.

4. Lice are small, flat wingless insects, divided into two groups: biting and sucking lice. They are most often found on a dog's neck and shoulders, especially behind the ears and under the collar.

5. The mosquito also bites with a syringelike mouth. Once a dog's skin is pierced, the mosquito's long probe sucks the dog's blood. During feeding, salivary fluids are introduced into the wound and cause irritation, itching, and swelling.

6. Flea and mosquito bites present other dangers to your dog's health. The most common tapeworm of dogs (and cats) uses the flea as its intermediate host. Most of the many varieties of mosquito can act as intermediate hosts of canine heartworm. (For more information, with suggestions for prevention and control, see "External Parasites" in section IV.)

Tick Bites

Ticks are bean-shaped and flat-bodied. Their size varies, but they can be as large as a kidney bean when fully engorged. Dogs are most often infested with two tick species: the brown dog tick and the American dog tick. Adult brown dog ticks are reddish brown and have four legs on each side of their bodies. When fully engorged, adult females turn a taupe color and appear rounded. American dog ticks are brown and have four legs on each side of their bodies. Adult males have mottled white areas on their top sides; females have a large white/cream-colored shield on their top sides immediately behind their heads. When fully engorged, adult females turn blue and appear rounded.

A tick bites by piercing the dog's skin and forcing its barbed mouth deep into the wound. As it sucks the dog's blood, the tick deposits salivary fluids in the wound; in this manner, disease can be transmitted to the animal. In addition to causing irritation and inflammation, tick bites can also result in anemia due to loss of blood.

Symptoms of Tick Bites

• Pain in affected area.

- Swelling under the skin.
- Usually the rear part of the tick is visible; it is often mistaken for a skin cyst.

Materials Required for Tick Bites

Tweezers or forceps
Alcohol, tick dip or spray
Antiseptic

Action for Tick Bites

1. Examine the dog's body thoroughly to locate all ticks. Check the insides of the ears, between the feet, under the front legs—the favorite hiding places.
2. Soak the ticks in alcohol or a small amount of tick spray, or coat them with petroleum jelly or mineral oil. This helps paralyze and asphyxiate the ticks and causes them to release their barbed-mouth grip. Wait 20 to 30 minutes and they should pull out easily.
3. Carefully remove each tick with a tweezers or forceps. If you use your fingers, shield your hand with a piece of paper. (See additional information at "External Parasites: Rocky Mountain spotted fever" in section IV.)
4. Do not twist the tick; pull it straight out. Be sure all parts are removed and that the head does not break off, remain in the skin, and cause infection.
5. After removing each tick, apply antiseptic to the area.
6. As soon as the ticks have been removed from the dog, burn them, flush them down the toilet, or drop them in alcohol. Do not crush them.
7. Wash your hands thoroughly with soap and water.

If there is a heavy infestation of ticks, see "External Parasites: Ticks" in section IV for additional information about control.

Bee, Hornet, Wasp, and Yellow-Jacket Stings and Ant Bites

These insects can present a serious problem, especially to dogs that are sensitive or allergic to their stings or venom.

Symptoms of Stings and Ant Bites

- Severe pain.
- After sting or bite, bitten part swells considerably. Stings on the face/head can be dangerous for Pugs, Boxers, Pekingese, Bulldogs, and other short-nosed breeds, as the swelling around the throat can cause added respiratory stress.
- Multiple stings may cause an acute allergic reaction and any or all of the following may occur:

1. Labored breathing.
2. Swelling of the tongue.
3. Salivation.
4. Dazed condition.
5. Collapse. (See "Allergy/Allergic Reactions.")

Materials Required for Stings and Ant Bites

Cold compress or ice
Tweezers or forceps
Insect sting relief
Antiseptic wipes/antiseptic

Emergency Action for Stings and Ant Bites

1. Assure a clear airway. Loosen the collar or anything tight around the dog's neck so that breathing is unobstructed.
2. Wipe affected area with antiseptic wipes.
3. If a stinger is visible, remove it with tweezers or forceps.
4. Activate instant cold compress or place some crushed ice in a plastic bag. Wrap either in a towel and apply to affected area for 5 to 10 minutes to help reduce swelling.
5. Apply insect sting relief.
6. *Watch for signs of acute allergic reaction.* If they occur or if the dog has experienced previous reaction to insect stings or bites, get to a veterinarian immediately. (See "Allergy/Allergic Reactions.")
7. If breathing stops, give artificial respiration en route. (See "Artificial Respiration.")

Bites from Poisonous Spiders (Black Widow, Brown Recluse, Common Brown) and Scorpion Stings

Spiders and scorpions are members of the class Arachnida. Arachnids are wingless and insectlike, with two body regions and 4 pairs of legs. Most arachnids in the United States are harmless, with the exception of the black widow spider, the brown recluse or "violin" spider, the common brown spider, and the scorpion.

Symptoms of Spider Bites and Scorpion Stings

* Swelling.
* Intense pain.
* Salivation.
* Difficulty in breathing.
* Nausea or vomiting.
* Open ulcer (brown recluse and common brown spider).
* Respiratory paralysis (scorpion).
* Convulsions (scorpion).
* Coma (scorpion).

Materials Required for Spider Bites and Scorpion Stings

Tweezers or forceps
Instant cold compress or ice
Antiseptic wipes or antiseptic

Emergency Action for Spider Bites and Scorpion Stings

1. Assure a clear airway. Loosen the collar or anything tight around the dog's neck so that breathing is unobstructed.
2. If breathing stops, start artificial respiration. (See "Artificial Respiration.")
3. If the bite is on a leg, apply a moderately tight tourniquet between the bite and the body to help stop the spread of venom.
4. Activate instant cold compress or place some crushed ice in a plastic bag. Wrap either in a towel and apply immediately above the bite.
5. Wipe the bite area with an antiseptic wipe or antiseptic.
6. Get the dog to a veterinarian immediately.
7. Treat for shock en route. (See "Shock.")

BITES AND STINGS FROM VENOMOUS ARACHNIDS

	Appearance	Biting or Stinging Mechanism	Symptoms
Black widow spiders	Only females are dangerous. Females have shiny black bodies with red markings, similar to an hourglass on the underside of the abdomen.	Black widow spiders bite their victims and inject venom from poison glands located on the chelicerae, or fanglike appendages. The glands are opened by a pore near the tip of each cheliceral fang.	Swelling and severe pain at site of bite. Nausea. Abdominal and muscle pains. Contraction of leg muscles. Respiratory difficulties. Elevated temperature.
Brown recluse or "violin" spider	Both males and females are dangerous. Generally yellowish brown with a darker mark on the top side. These spiders are shaped broader in front and narrower behind, resembling a violin.	Brown recluse spiders bite their victims and inject venom from poison glands located on the chelicerae, or fanglike appendages. These glands are opened by a pore near the tip of each cheliceral fang.	The bite itself may be painless but tenderness and redness will appear a few hours later. Within 24 hours, the victim will experience nausea, chills, and elevated temperature. Reaction from venom can cause the formation of an open ulcer in 7–12 days, which is slow to heal.
Scorpion	Pale salmon color. Two body regions and four pairs of legs. Scorpions have long segmented tails that end in a sting.	Venom is injected into victim through a stinger which is located at the base of the scorpion's tail. When feeding, restricted, or distressed, the scorpion will raise its tail and strike, forcing its sting into the victim.	Symptoms of a scorpion sting depend on the species of scorpion; amount of venom injected; age, size, and physical condition of victim, but include severe pain; discoloration and swelling at site of sting; restlessness; nausea; vomiting; respiratory paralysis; abdominal pains; convulsions; shock and coma.

INSECTICIDES, OVEREXPOSURE TO

If your dog has swallowed, inhaled, or absorbed an insecticide through its skin, see "Poisoning." For common-sense information about using flea collars and insecticidal sprays and dips, see "External Parasites" in Section IV.

ITCHING AND SCRATCHING

Many conditions can cause severe itching and scratching. See "Allergy/Allergic Reactions," "External Parasites" in Section IV, and "Skin Problems" in Section IV.

MOTION SICKNESS

Many dogs experience motion sickness when they ride in cars or other moving vehicles. Overfeeding (too much food or water beforehand), fear or excitement at being confined, lack of fresh air, or the speeding up or slowing down of a vehicle can cause nausea and vomiting. Young dogs seem to be most susceptible to motion sickness; they tend to outgrow this tendency as they mature.

Prevention

The best prevention is to allow your dog to gain car experience in gradual stages. Whatever your life-style—city, suburban, or country—try to fit your dog's car training into your daily schedule. Start by making short, frequent trips. Go shopping, chauffeur the children, or just take a drive, but make each little excursion a pleasant experience for the pet. Use the following guidelines to help with car training:

1. Don't give solid food for 8 hours before the trip. Allow a limited amount of water.
2. Before getting in the car, give the dog time to urinate or have a bowel movement.

3. Cover the car seat with newspapers or towels. Weather permitting, allow good ventilation. While the vehicle is in motion, let the dog look through the window if it is inquisitive but *not to put its head outside*. A dog that is known to get carsick should not be allowed to move all over the car. In case of vomiting, it's less messy to clean up a small area instead of half the car. Confine the dog to a restricted area by tying its lead to one of the seat belts. (However, never tie the dog or leave its lead on when it is alone in the car.) This is also a good way to control a disobedient puppy whose excessive jumping could be dangerous to the driver.

4. As previously mentioned, if you notice panting or excessive drooling, stop the car in a safe place, get out and let the dog stretch its legs.

5. Eventually, as the dog becomes accustomed to a variety of situations in a moving vehicle, fear and anxiety should pass and the dog will become a veteran traveler.

6. If necessary, use a nonnarcotic calmative for dogs to help control motion sickness. Such products are available at most pet stores and usually are given to the dog about 30 minutes before departure. Follow the manufacturer's directions carefully. If your dog turns out to be one of the few that cannot ride without becoming nauseated, a veterinarian can prescribe preventive medication. Pay attention to your dog's behavior, describe any symptoms or reactions to your veterinarian, and let him prescribe necessary medication to help control the problem.

Symptoms

- Restlessness.
- Panting or excessive salivation (drooling).
- Vomiting.
- Diarrhea (not always present).

Materials Required for Action

A supply of newspapers
Towels and damp washcloth
Nonnarcotic motion sickness preparation for pets

Action

1. Prepare in advance by covering the car seat with newspapers.
2. When riding, if the dog starts to swallow or drool excessively, stop the car in a safe place. Attach the dog's collar and lead. Get out of the car and let the pet exercise and breathe fresh air.
3. Use towels and a damp washcloth to clean up the dog and the car if vomiting occurs.

PARALYSIS

Paralysis has a number of causes, including fracture of the vertebral column (spine), spinal cord injury, ruptures or degeneration of intervertebral disks, brain tumors or injuries, and nerve damage from serious injuries, canine distemper, rabies, and some kinds of poisoning. Depending on the location and type of injury, there may be other serious complications. Any partial or total loss of feeling or movement requires the immediate attention of a veterinarian.

Symptoms

- Loss of feeling in one or more legs.
- Dragging hindquarters.
- Dog unable to support weight on legs.
- Partial loss of facial muscles (excessive salivation, sagging eyelids).
- Breathing difficulties.

Materials Required for Emergency Action

Blanket
Firm, flat surface for transportation

Emergency Action

1. Keep air passages clear. Loosen the collar or anything tight around the neck that might obstruct breathing.

2. If breathing stops, administer artificial respiration. (See "Artificial Respiration.")
3. Handle the dog with great care to prevent additional damage.
4. Place the dog on a flat, firm surface for transportation. Move the body carefully, following the instructions in "Emergency Transportation of Injured Dogs."
5. Keep the dog warm and quiet.
6. Get to a veterinarian immediately.
7. Recovery from paralysis is slow, and much love, patience, and competent home nursing will be necessary. Consult Section II, "Home Nursing."

POISONING

DOGS CAN BE POISONED:

1. By mouth (swallowing poison)
2. Through the skin (absorbing poison)
3. By inhaling (exposure to fumes, smoke, gases)

Many cases of dog poisoning are accidental and caused by human ignorance or carelessness. Pet owners often fail to keep toxic substances out of reach of their pets, allowing them access to spoiled food or garbage, or they do not read labels correctly when mixing insecticides or pesticides. Sadly, there are people who will deliberately poison a dog; this too is often the fault of the dog's owner because the pet has been allowed to wander and become the neighborhood nuisance.

Dogs, especially young puppies, are much like children, full of curiosity and tempted to chew anything they can get into their mouths. Some dogs that are left alone a great deal or have nothing interesting to do (such as playing with safe toys or regular exercise periods) chew and swallow toxic materials and objects out of boredom.

Because there are so many common indoor and outdoor items that can poison a dog, try to be a concerned pet owner and take time to become aware of all potential poisoning hazards. If you have not yet completed your dog's Medical Record chart at the beginning of section IV, do it now. *Record the telephone numbers of your veterinarian and Poison Control Center now.*

Household Hazards

Every room in the house contains items that can produce toxic reactions in dogs. Any product identified as being dangerous or poisonous to children or adults also will be toxic for pets. You can help prevent accidental poisoning by keeping all potentially toxic substances out of your dog's reach.

LAUNDRY ROOM
Detergent
Soap
Water softener
Bleach (powdered and liquid)
Spot remover/cleaning solution
Fabric dye

KITCHEN
Dishwashing compound
Scouring pad
Disinfectant, sanitizer
Cleaning and polishing product for furniture, walls, or floors
Silver polish or cream
Ammonia
Drain cleaner
Oven cleaner
Metal cleaner and polish
Ant and roach spray and other insecticides
Diet pills
Scouring powder

BEDROOM
Sleeping pills
Birth-control pills
Contraceptive cream
Mothballs and other antimoth products
Cigarettes

BATHROOM
Laxative

Nail polish/polish remover
Toilet bowl cleaner
Drain opener
Rubbing alcohol
Deodorant and antiperspirant
Product for athlete's foot
Tranquilizer
Sleeping pills
Liniment
Suntan lotion
Certain cosmetics and toiletries. Keep those labeled "For
    External Use Only" out of the dog's reach
Certain bath preparations
Certain after-shave lotions/perfumes
Shampoo
Headache remedy
Hair dye/rinse/bleach

GARAGE
Antifreeze
Brake fluid
Radiator cleaner
Carburetor cleaner
Gasoline
Kerosene
Rust/corrosion inhibitor
Battery
Insecticide
Chlorine swimming-pool preparation

BASEMENT
Paint
Paint and varnish remover
Wax
Polish
Paint thinner
Solvent
Calking compounds
Brush cleaner
Pesticide
Fungicide
Fertilizer
Insecticide
Bulbs, seeds, plants
Shoe polish

Charcoal starter
Cleaning fluid

HOBBY ROOM OR WORKSHOP
Photographic developer/fixative
Antiquing products
Oil paint
Tempera paint
Lead-based paint
Lacquer thinner
Glue
Preservative
Green or purple ink
Marking crayons (children's crayons are nontoxic)
Indelible pencils

Note: Some of the items listed here are highly toxic and not meant to be ingested. Others may seem harmless; however, when eaten in large amount, they can prove hazardous or even fatal to your dog.

Swallowed Poisons

Symptoms of swallowed poisons are always dose- and time-related. Early signs can vary and make accurate diagnosis difficult; therefore, even if you only suspect that your dog has eaten something toxic, don't wait for signs to appear. Seek veterinary help immediately, for *speed may be necessary to save your dog's life.* The degree of tolerance to a poison depends on a dog's age and general health, as well as the amount ingested. Young puppies or older dogs are more vulnerable to severe poisoning, and a small amount of poison can kill a weak or debilitated pet.

Dogs can become poisoned by swallowing drugs, pesticides, insecticides, chemicals, and other household substances. The toxic substances chart lists some common potentially toxic substances and their emergency treatment.

COMMON TOXIC SUBSTANCES:
SOURCES, SIGNS OF TOXICITY, AND EMERGENCY TREATMENT

	Sources	Signs of Toxicity[a]	Treatment[b]
Amphetamines	Diet and pep pills	*Mild:* Restlessness; dilated pupils; insomnia; *Severe:* Convulsions; coma; death	INDUCE vomiting immediately. Dilute remaining poison with milk or water. Consult veterinarian. Recovery depends on amount ingested and early treatment.
Arsenic	Insecticides; herbicides; certain paints; ant and rat poisons;	Highly toxic with rapid onset of symptoms. Salivation; vomiting; watery diarrhea (often bloody); severe abdominal pain; garliclike odor of vomitus; dehydration; coma; shock; death	INDUCE vomiting. Dilute remaining poison with milk or beaten egg white. See veterinarian immediately. Treatment effective if started early.
Ethylene glycol	Antifreeze; Sterno; windshield deicer (dogs are attracted to its sweet taste)	Vomiting; progressive depression; delirium; convulsions; coma; death	INDUCE vomiting. Dilute remaining poison with milk. *Highly toxic. Get to a veterinarian immediately. Pet may survive if treated early.*
Lead	Lead-based paints; putty; golf balls;	Profuse salivation; vomiting; loss of appetite; abdominal	INDUCE vomiting. Give activated charcoal. See veteri-

	pesticides; some linoleums; batteries (lead poisoning can occur at any age but teething or curious puppies 2–7 months old are very susceptible)	pain; progressive depression; bloating; sensitivity to light; convulsions	narian for treatment. Fatal if not treated promptly.
Thallium	Rodent poisons; some depilatory creams	Signs may not appear immediately, but 1–3 days after ingestion: vomiting; black diarrhea; weakness; loss of appetite; depression. Skin appears "brick red" 2–4 days after exposure and may become ulcerated. As condition progresses: muscle twitching; convulsions; coma	INDUCE vomiting. Dilute remaining poison with milk or water. Consult veterinarian immediately; for survival depends on early treatment.

[a] Symptoms are always dose- and time-related. Early signs can be nonspecific and make accurate diagnosis complex. If you think your dog may have ingested something toxic, don't wait for signs to appear. Seek veterinary help immediately.

[b] See more detailed treatment under "Poisoning: Swallowed Poisons." If a veterinarian cannot be reached, call your local Poison Control Center for help.

	Sources	Signs of Toxicity[a]	Treatment[b]
Strychnine	Rodent poisons	Highly toxic with rapid onset of signs: dilated pupils; excessive thirst; salivation; violent convulsions (the slightest noise, touch, or bright lights will cause the animal to convulse)	DO NOT INDUCE vomiting. Dilute the poison with large quantities of milk or water. Get to veterinarian immediately. Keep warm and quiet en route to discourage seizures.
Sodium Fluoroacetate (Compond 1080)	Rodent poisons	Highly toxic. May be inhaled, swallowed, or absorbed through skin. Rapid onset of symptoms: vomiting; panting; nervousness; repeated urination and diarrhea; violent convulsions; death	INDUCE vomiting immediately. Dilute remaining poison with large amounts of milk or water. No known antidote. Get to veterinarian for treatment immediately.
ANTU (Alpha-naphthyl thiourea)	Rodent poisons	Highly toxic with rapid onset of signs: vomiting; diarrhea; stomach upset; difficult breathing; pulmonary edema. As condition progresses, dog almost drowns from fluid buildup in its lungs. Restlessness; collapse; death	INDUCE vomiting immediately. Dilute remaining poison with large amounts of milk or water. No specific antidote. Consult veterinarian immediately. Treatment must be started as soon as possible.

Warfarin (D-Con) and other anticoagulant rodenticides such as Pindone and Diphacinone	Rodent poisons	These are anticoagulants and interfere with normal clotting factors, causing hemorrhage; pale mucous membranes; bloody stool; difficult breathing; progressive depression; weakness; lameness; convulsions; death	INDUCE vomiting immediately. Dilute remaining poison with large amounts of milk or water. Consult veterinarian immediately for oxygen therapy and blood transfusions.
Petroleum distillates	Gasoline; kerosene; paint thinner; paint remover; lighter fluid	Nausea; vomiting; breathing difficulties; pulmonary edema; dizziness; weakness; loss of consciousness; convulsions	DO NOT INDUCE vomiting. Dilute poison with milk or beaten egg whites. See veterinarian immediately.
Organophosphates and carbamate insecticides	Insecticides such as: Dichlorvos (DDVP, Vapona); Ronnel; Malathion; Diazinon; Fenthion;	Extremely toxic. Exposure can be oral, through skin or by inhalation, causing salivation; muscle twitching; vomiting; diarrhea; difficult breathing;	INDUCE vomiting immediately. Dilute remaining poison with large amounts of milk or water. Specific antidotes available. Consult veterinarian

[a] Symptoms are always dose- and time-related. Early signs can be nonspecific and make accurate diagnosis complex. If you think your dog may have ingested something toxic, don't wait for signs to appear. Seek veterinary help immediately.

[b] See more detailed treatment under "Poisoning: Swallowed Poisons." If a veterinarian cannot be reached, call your local Poison Control Center for help.

	Sources	Signs of Toxicity[a]	Treatment[b]
	Dimethoate; and Imidran	constricted pupils; paralysis; convulsions; coma; death	immediately. Skin exposure: wash immediately with warm water and shampoo. Dry and keep warm.
Chlorinated hydrocarbons	Insecticides such as DDT, Lindane, Chlordane, Aldrin, Endrin, Benzene, Dieldrin, Hexachloride, and Toxaphene (pets become exposed by walking or lying on contaminated surfaces; poisoning can also occur by pet licking coat or paws)	Exposure can be oral or through the skin, causing depression; muscle twitching; convulsions; high temperature during and following seizures (the slightest noise, touch, or bright light may cause a seizure); coma; death	INDUCE vomiting immediately if dog is not convulsing. Be careful when giving emetic, as this could cause a seizure and cause the dog to inhale its vomitus. DO NOT GIVE milk or oil; GIVE activated charcoal or water to dilute. Consult veterinarian immediately. Skin exposure: wash with soap and water. Dry and keep warm.
Phenol (carbolic acid)	Some disinfecting products; wood preservatives; fungicides; herbicides; some photograph developers	Exposure can be oral or through the skin, causing abdominal pain; pale skin and mucous membranes; nausea; vomiting; incoordination; depression	INDUCE vomiting immediately. Dilute remaining poison with olive oil or activated charcoal. No antidote available. See veterinarian immediately for medical treatment.

		Skin exposure: wash with soap and water. Dry and keep warm.
Metaldehyde	Snail and slug poisons (dogs are often attracted to these products)	Poisoning occurs most often in climates where snails and slugs are prevalent. Symptoms include anxiety; salivation; convulsions. The seizures are continuous and not influenced by noise, touch, or bright lights as in strychnine or chlorinated hydrocarbon poisoning.	INDUCE vomiting immediately. Be careful when giving emetic as this could initiate a seizure and cause dog to inhale vomitus into lungs. Dilute remaining poison with milk or water. See veterinarian immediately for treatment.
Phosphorus (white or yellow)	Some rodent poisons; fireworks; "strike-anywhere" matches; striking surfaces of matchbooks	Abdominal pain; vomiting; diarrhea; staggering gait; breath and vomitus with a garlic odor; progressive nervousness; collapse; coma; death[l]	INDUCE vomiting immediately. DO NOT GIVE milk or oil to dilute remaining poison; GIVE only activated charcoal in water. Consult veterinarian immediately.

---

[a] Symptoms are always dose- and time-related. Early signs can be nonspecific and make accurate diagnosis complex. If you think your dog may have ingested something toxic, don't wait for signs to appear. Seek veterinary help immediately.

[b] See more detailed treatment under "Poisoning: Swallowed Poisons." If a veterinarian cannot be reached, call your local Poison Control Center for help.

	Sources	Signs of Toxicity[a]	Treatment[b]
Barbiturates	Sleeping pills; sedatives	Staggering gait; drowsiness; shock; coma; death	INDUCE vomiting immediately. Administer stimulant: warm strong coffee or tea. Keep dog awake and moving. Consult veterinarian immediately.
Garbage and food poisons	Access to spoiled food	Nausea; vomiting; severe abdominal pain; bloated abdomen; diarrhea; staggering gait; shock	INDUCE vomiting immediately. If abdomen is greatly swollen, use disposable enema to help empty colon. Consult veterinarian immediately.
Nicotine	Cigarettes (dogs most often poisoned after eating large amounts); nicotine in cigarette filters	Salivation; pale mucous membranes; severe depression; breathing difficulties; vomiting; eating large amounts can cause respiratory distress	INDUCE vomiting immediately. Dilute remaining amount with activated charcoal and water. See veterinarian immediately. Give artificial respiration if breathing stops.
Acetylsalicylic acid, salicylates	Aspirin	Vomiting; panting; breath may smell like nail polish remover; convulsions; collapse	INDUCE vomiting immediately. Dilute remaining amount with milk or water.

144

Poison	Sources	Symptoms	What to do
			See veterinarian immediately.
Acids (acetic, hydrochloric, nitric, sulfuric, etc.)	Household bleaches; some metal cleaners and polishes; certain disinfectants; car batteries (sulfuric acid); chlorine swimming pool preparations	Burning pain in mouth; yellowish or brownish stains around mouth; vomiting (often bloodstained); severe abdominal pain; muscle tremors; weak pulse; rapid, shallow breathing; collapse	The principal effect of acid poisoning is corrosion. DO NOT INDUCE vomiting. DILUTE the acid as quickly as possible with large quantities of milk, beaten egg whites, or water. (Do not waste time, as a delay of only a few minutes can severely damage the esophagus and stomach.) Then give milk of magnesia to neutralize the acid. Get dog to veterinarian immediately.
Alkalies (weak)	Soaps; dishwashing detergents; laundry detergents; shampoos	Nausea; vomiting; diarrhea	INDUCE vomiting immediately. Give large amounts of milk or water. See veterinarian immediately.

^a Symptoms are always dose- and time-related. Early signs can be nonspecific and make accurate diagnosis complex. If you think your dog may have ingested something toxic, don't wait for signs to appear. Seek veterinary help immediately.

^b See more detailed treatment under "Poisoning: Swallowed Poisons." If a veterinarian cannot be reached, call your local Poison Control Center for help.

	Sources	Signs of Toxicity[a]	Treatment[b]
Alkalies (strong): sodium hydroxide (lye); potassium hydroxide; sodium phosphates; ammonium hydroxide	Ammonia; drain cleaners; grease dissolvers; caustic soda; water softeners; some polishes and cleaning products	Severe abdominal pain; vomiting (often bloodstained); diarrhea; collapse	The principal effect of alkali poisoning is corrosion. DO NOT INDUCE vomiting. DILUTE the alkali as quickly as possible with milk or water. (Don't waste time, as a delay of a few minutes can cause severe damage.) Then give 2–3 tablespoons vinegar or lemon juice (fresh or bottled) mixed with equal parts water to neutralize the alkali. Get to veterinarian immediately.

[a] Symptoms are always dose- and time-related. Early signs can be nonspecific and make accurate diagnosis complex. If you think your dog may have ingested something toxic, don't wait for signs to appear. Seek veterinary help immediately.
[b] See more detailed treatment under "Poisoning: Swallowed Poisons." If a veterinarian cannot be reached, call your local Poison Control Center for help.

Today, because of a general interest in gardening and houseplants, dogs come into contact with many plant varieties. Most plants are harmless, but there are over 700 types of plants in this hemisphere which can be potentially toxic (even deadly) to dogs. Because many pets nibble on house or garden plants, it is sensible to learn which varieties can be dangerous.

If you think your dog has eaten a poisonous plant, call your veterinarian or Poison Control Center immediately to determine if vomiting should be induced. Ingestion of certain plants causes burning and irritation and swelling of the mouth and tongue; in this case vomiting should not be induced. The hazardous plants chart list some plants that are dangerous to dogs, the toxic parts of the plants, and some general signs of toxicity.

HAZARDOUS COMMON HOUSE AND GARDEN PLANTS

	Toxic Part	Signs of Toxicity
House plants:		
Alocasia[a]	All parts	Burning, irritation, and swelling of mouth and tongue; salivation
Bird of paradise	All parts	Immediate nausea; vomiting; diarrhea; abdominal pain
Caladium[a]	Leaves, roots	Burning, irritation, and swelling of mouth and tongue; salivation; difficult breathing; vomiting
Castor beans	Seeds	Burning of mouth and throat; excessive thirst; stomach pains; diarrhea

[a] Especially dangerous because death can result if base of tongue swells enough to block air passage to the throat.

[b] Do not leave unplanted bulbs in garage or basement where dogs can reach them.

	Toxic Part	Signs of Toxicity
Dumb cane[a] (Dieffenbachia)	All parts	Burning, irritation, and swelling of mouth and tongue; excessive salivation
Elephant's ear[a]	All parts	Burning, irritation, and swelling of mouth and tongue; salivation
Jequirity bean	Seeds	May be fatal. Chills; abdominal pains; irregular pulse
Mistletoe	Berries	Can be fatal. Acute stomach and intestinal irritation; weakened pulse; diarrhea
Mother-in-law	Leaves	Enzyme produces swelling of the tongue
Philodendron[a]	All parts	Burning, irritation, and swelling of mouth and tongue; salivation
Poinsettia	Leaves, sap, stem	*Leaves and stem:* severe irritation to mouth, throat, and stomach. Can be fatal. *Sap:* causes skin irritation and, if rubbed into eyes, can cause severe irritation
Precatory bean Rosary pea	Seeds	Can be fatal. Chills; depression
Skunk cabbage[a]	All parts	Burning, irritation, and swelling of mouth and tongue; salivation

[a] Especially dangerous because death can result if base of tongue swells enough to block air passage to the throat.

[b] Do not leave unplanted bulbs in garage or basement where dogs can reach them.

	Toxic Part	Signs of Toxicity
Garden and ornamental plants:		
Amaryllis[b]	Bulb	Immediate nausea; vomiting; diarrhea
Azalea	All parts	Nausea; vomiting; progressive depression; staggering gait; breathing difficulties
Bleeding heart (Dutchman's-breeches)	Foliage, roots	When eaten in large amounts can cause breathing difficulties and convulsions
Buttercup	All parts	Stomach irritation; diarrhea; convulsions when eaten in large quantities
Cactus	All parts	Abscesses; mouth irritations; hemorrhage; lameness
Chinaberry	All parts	Convulsions
Christmas rose	Rootstalks, leaves	Skin inflammation; numbing of mouth tissues; stomach upset; nervousness
Crocus, autumn	All parts	Vomiting; nervous excitement
Crown of thorns	All parts	Irritating sap causes severe inflammation of mouth, throat, and stomach if swallowed
Daffodil[b]	Bulb	Can be fatal. Nausea; vomiting; diarrhea; diges-

---

[a] Especially dangerous because death can result if base of tongue swells enough to block air passage to the throat.

[b] Do not leave unplanted bulbs in garage or basement where dogs can reach them.

149

	Toxic Part	Signs of Toxicity
		tive upsets; trembling; chills
Daphne	Berries, leaves, bark	Digestive upsets; abdominal pain; vomiting; bloody diarrhea; weakness; convulsions
Delphinium	Seeds, young plants	Toxicity increases with plant's age. Digestive upsets; nervous excitement and depression when eaten in large quantities
Four-o'clock	Roots, seeds	Powdered root causes irritation of throat and skin
Foxglove	Leaves, seeds	Can be fatal. Cardiovascular disturbances; irregular heartbeat and pulse; immediate nausea; confusion
Golden chain	Beanlike capsules which contain seeds	Can be fatal. Nausea; excitement; staggering gait; poisoning; convulsions; coma
Holly	Berries	Salivation; vomiting; diarrhea; abdominal pain; collapse
Hyacinth[b]	Bulb	Can be fatal. Nausea; vomiting; diarrhea
Hydrangea	All parts	Vomiting; breathing difficulties; coma

---

[a] Especially dangerous because death can result if base of tongue swells enough to block air passage to the throat.
[b] Do not leave unplanted bulbs in garage or basement where dogs can reach them.

	Toxic Part	Signs of Toxicity
Iris (blue flag)	Under-ground stems, leaves	Immediate nausea; abdominal pain; diarrhea
Ivy, English	All parts	Salivation; immediate nausea; difficulty in breathing; diarrhea; abdominal pain; collapse
Jerusalem cherry	All parts (especially berries, which contain a toxic alkaloid)	Can be fatal. Rapid pulse; dilated pupils; excessive thirst; digestive upset
Jessamine, yellow	Berries	Can be fatal. Rapid pulse; dilated pupils; excessive thirst; digestive upset
Jonquil[b]	Bulb	Nausea; vomiting; diarrhea; causes convulsions if eaten in large amounts
Lantana	All parts	Can be fatal. Affects lungs, heart, kidney, and nervous system, causing muscular weakness and stomach irritation
Larkspur	Seeds, young plants	Can be fatal. Nervousness; digestive upset; progressive depression
Laurel, mountain	All parts	Can be fatal. Salivation; vomiting; staggering gait; breathing difficulties; convulsions

---

[a] Especially dangerous because death can result if base of tongue swells enough to block air passage to the throat.

[b] Do not leave unplanted bulbs in garage or basement where dogs can reach them.

151

	Toxic Part	Signs of Toxicity
Lily, calla	All parts	Can be fatal if base of tongue swells and blocks passage of air. Irritation and swelling of mouth, tongue and throat; breathing difficulties
Lily, climbing or glory	All parts	Nervous excitement; serious digestive upset; diarrhea
Lily of the valley	Leaves, flowers	Cardiovascular disturbances; irregular heartbeat and pulse; immediate nausea; confusion
Monkshood	All parts	Immediate nausea; nervous excitement; tremors; convulsions
Morning glory	Seeds	Produces LSD-like effects; can cause death from severe mental disturbances
Narcissus[b]	Bulb	Nausea; vomiting; diarrhea
Oleander	Leaves, branches	Cardiovascular disturbances; irregular heartbeat and pulse; dizziness; Immediate nausea; serious digestive upset
Peony	Roots	Juice may cause paralysis
Privet, common	All parts	Immediate nausea; stomach irritation; nervousness; diarrhea
Rhododendron	All parts	Can be fatal. Nausea; vomiting; breathing diffi-

[a] Especially dangerous because death can result if base of tongue swells enough to block air passage to the throat.
[b] Do not leave unplanted bulbs in garage or basement where dogs can reach them.

	Toxic Part	Signs of Toxicity
		culties; staggering gait; collapse; coma
Snowdrop[b]	All parts (especially bulb)	Digestive upset; general nervous excitement
Star-of-Bethlehem[b]	Bulb	Vomiting; nervous excitement
Sweet pea	Stem	Can be fatal. Stem can cause a type of paralysis
Tobacco	Leaves	Salivation; immediate nausea; rapid heartbeat
Violet (pansy)	Seeds	Laxative effects can be serious when eaten in large quantities
Virginia creeper	All parts	Can be fatal. Delayed vomiting; abdominal pain; progressive depression; coma
Wisteria	Seeds, pods	Immediate nausea; mild to serious digestive upset; abdominal pain
Yew	Seeds, foliage, bark	Can be fatal. Immediate nausea; vomiting; abdominal pain; diarrhea; convulsions. Contains an alkaloid which depresses heart action
Trees and shrubs:		
Apple	Seeds	Can be fatal. When eaten in large quantities, can cause cyanide poisoning

[a] Especially dangerous because death can result if base of tongue swells enough to block air passage to the throat.

[b] Do not leave unplanted bulbs in garage or basement where dogs can reach them.

	Toxic Part	Signs of Toxicity
Apricot	Pits	When eaten in large amounts may cause coma. Vomiting; breathing difficulties
Black locust	Bark, sprouts, foliage, seeds	Immediate nausea; weakness; progressive depression
Cherry	Leaves, twigs, seeds, tree bark	Can be fatal: contains a compound which releases cyanide when ingested, causing breathing difficulties; nervous excitement; collapse
Elderberry	All parts (especially roots)	Nausea; vomiting; digestive upset
Oak	Foliage, acorns	Gradually affects kidneys but requires a large amount to be toxic
Peach	Leaves, pits, tree bark	Can be fatal: contains a compound which releases cyanide when ingested, causing breathing difficulties; nervous excitement; collapse
Pine	Needles	Not toxic but included because serious reaction can occur if needles are eaten.

[a] Especially dangerous because death can result if base of tongue swells enough to block air passage to the throat.
[b] Do not leave unplanted bulbs in garage or basement where dogs can reach them.

	Toxic Part	Signs of Toxicity
Garden vegetable plants:		
Potato	Foliage, sprouts, green parts	Normal potatoes are harmless when eaten in large amounts. However, there is potential danger in the green spots of the tubers, in sprouts or in decomposing potatoes. These should not be fed to dogs
Rhubarb	Leaves, blades	The leaf stalk which is normally eaten is harmless but the blade contains acids that can be hazardous when large quantities are ingested. Eating large amounts of raw or cooked leaves can cause nervousness; convulsions; coma
Tomato	Green parts	When eaten in large amounts can cause cardiac depression
Wild plants:		
Baneberry	All parts	Immediate nausea; vomiting; diarrhea; intestinal upset
Bittersweet	Leaves, unripe fruit	Delayed nausea and vomiting; abdominal pain; diarrhea
Buckeye (horse chestnut)	All parts	Immediate nausea and vomiting; abdominal pain; diarrhea

[a] Especially dangerous because death can result if base of tongue swells enough to block air passage to the throat.

[b] Do not leave unplanted bulbs in garage or basement where dogs can reach them.

155

	Toxic Part	Signs of Toxicity
Buttercup	All parts	Irritating juices can cause serious digestive upset
Hemlock, poison	All parts	Can be fatal. Excessive salivation; immediate vomiting; digestive disturbances; rapid heartbeat
Hemlock, water (cowbane)	All parts	Can be fatal. Diarrhea; collapse; convulsions
Jack-in-the-pulpit	All parts	Can be fatal if base of tongue swells enough to stop air passage. Irritation, burning, and swelling of mouth and tongue; excess salivation
Jimsonweed (thornapple)	All parts	Excessive thirst; dry mouth tissues; difficult or labored breathing; rapid heartbeat and pulse
Laurel	All parts	Salivation; vomiting; staggering gait; breathing difficulties; convulsions
Marsh marigold	All parts	Irritation of mouth and tongue; digestive upset; breathing difficulties; diarrhea; convulsions
Moonseed	Berries: blue or purple in color, resembling wild grapes	Severe digestive upset; abdominal pain

[a] Especially dangerous because death can result if base of tongue swells enough to block air passage to the throat.
[b] Do not leave unplanted bulbs in garage or basement where dogs can reach them.

	Toxic Part	Signs of Toxicity
Mushroom (fly agaric and amanita group)	All parts	Can be fatal. Excessive thirst; severe abdominal pain; breathing difficulties
Nightshade	All parts	Can be fatal. Severe digestive disturbances
Poison ivy, oak, or sumac	All parts	Severe itching and scratching; blistered skin. Usually dogs do not eat these plants, but they can get oil on their coats which may produce these symptoms
Pokeweed	All parts	Immediate vomiting; severe abdominal pain; diarrhea

[a] Especially dangerous because death can result if base of tongue swells enough to block air passage to the throat.

[b] Do not leave unplanted bulbs in garage or basement where dogs can reach them.

Recommended reading for additional information about potentially hazardous plants:

Kingsbury, John M.: *Common Poisonous Plants*. Cornell University Extension Bulletin 538, Ithaca, N.Y.

Kingsbury, John M.: *Deadly Harvest: A Guide to Common Poisonous Plants*.

Lampe, K. F., and Fagerstrom, R.: *Plant Toxicity and Dermatitis: A Manual for Physicians*.

Muenscher, Walter C.: *Poisonous Plants of the United States*.

Typical Poisonous Plants. Pamphlet, U.S. Health Service.

PRIME OBJECTIVES IN TREATING DOGS
THAT HAVE SWALLOWED POISONS

1. Induce vomiting, which removes the poison from the body and decreases absorption and damage.
2. Dilute the poison if it cannot be vomited and help delay further absorption.
3. Get your dog at once to a veterinarian for antidote and medical treatment.

Materials Required for Swallowed Poisons

Emetic to induce vomiting (see below)
Milk, beaten egg whites, vegetable oil, or Milk of Bismuth
Activated charcoal
Blanket

Emergency Action for Swallowed Poisons

Do not administer first aid if the dog is convulsing or unconscious—seek veterinary help immediately.

1. Call a veterinarian at once. If you cannot reach your regular veterinarian, call any nearby one. Give as much information as you can over the phone so the veterinarian can help by giving instructions for appropriate treatment. If possible, have another person make the call while you begin first aid.
2. Give an emetic to induce vomiting. *(Before administering emetic, read step 3.)* Use one of the following mixtures:
   a. 3% Hydrogen Peroxide. Give undiluted or mix with equal parts water (1–2 tablespoonsful per 10 pounds of body weight).
   b. 1 tablespoonful ordinary table salt dissolved in 1 cup of warm water.
   c. 1 tablespoonful powdered mustard dissolved in 1 cup of warm water.

   Pour the liquid into the side of the dog's mouth, using the lip-pocket method. (See "How to Give Medicines:

158

Giving Liquids by the 'Lip-Pocket Method' " in section II.) Repeat in 5 to 8 minutes if vomiting does not occur. (Save a sample of the dog's vomitus in a plastic bag for the veterinarian's identification.)

3. *Do not induce vomiting* if the dog has swallowed corrosive acid or alkali, kerosene, gasoline or other petroleum distillates, or strychnine. Making the dog vomit would burn the esophagus. Instead, dilute the poison to delay further absorption by giving quantities of milk, beaten egg whites, vegetable oil, or Milk of Bismuth. If nothing else is available immediately, use water, as it will increase the amount of fluid which must be absorbed for a given amount of poison.

4. *Get the dog to a veterinarian at once.* If you have phoned in advance, the veterinarian can be prepared to give immediate treatment.

5. If you are unable to reach a veterinarian within a short time and the poison can be identified, check to see if a specific antidote is listed on the package or call your local Poison Control Center* for information. If you do not know or own the specific antidote, mix 3 to 4 tablespoons of activated charcoal in 1 cup of water or milk (double the amount for large breeds) and give to the dog by the lip-pocket method to help prevent further absorption. Then proceed to the veterinary hospital as soon as possible.

6. Try to keep the dog warm and quiet en route. Remember that certain poisons cause convulsions and the slightest noise, touch, or light may cause the dog to have a seizure. Wrap the dog in a towel or blanket to prevent further injury. Try to keep the head lower than the body to allow fluids to run out of the mouth.

7. Watch for respiratory distress. If breathing stops, start artifical respiration. (See "Artificial Respiration.")

8. Treat for shock. (See "Shock.")

---

* Poison control centers in the United States and Canada have been established to inform physicians and veterinarians as well as individuals about the toxicities of commercial products, medicines, insecticides, pesticides, etc. All significant data on the toxic ingredients in hundreds of thousands of products are on file in these centers.

Skin Contact Poisons

Skin contact with poisons can be caused by the dog walking, rolling, or lying on contaminated surfaces or by accidental spilling of burning or corrosive substances on its skin and coat.

Symptoms of Skin Contact Poisons

- Redness and/or rash.
- Pain
- Mild to severe skin reactions.
- Skin peeling.
- Loss of hair (not always).

Emergency Action for Skin Contact Poisons

1. Flush the skin, using a shower spray or hose, with large amounts of lukewarm water to remove any unabsorbed materials. If the eyes are involved, flush with warm water under low pressure, holding the lids apart. *Eye contact requires the immediate attention of a veterinarian.* (See "Eye Emergencies.")
2. If the substance contained an alkali, rinse or sponge the skin with equal parts of vinegar and water. Do not apply before water flushing or you may burn the dog's skin. Do not get mixture in the eyes.
3. If the substance contained acid, mix 3 to 4 tablespoons of baking soda and 1 quart of warm water and rinse or sponge on the dog's skin. Do not apply before water flushing.
4. For gasoline, kerosene, petroleum distillates, or solvent distillates (paint thinners), saturate the dog with vegetable oil or milk. Twenty to 30 minutes later, wash the oil or milk out of the coat with shampoo and water, rinse thoroughly, and dry. Vegetable oil can be difficult to remove from the coat; if a large amount was necessary for saturation, try using a gentle liquid dish detergent (Liquid Lux, Ivory, etc.) to wash it out of the hair.
5. To remove latex paint, wash the dog with shampoo and water. Rinse thoroughly and dry. Repeat if necessary.
6. To remove oil-based paints, let the paint dry on the

coat. Then clip or scissor off as much paint-covered hair as possible. Soak any remaining areas with vegetable oil. Wipe the coat with an old terry towel and repeat the oil soakings until the paint begins to loosen. Then bathe with shampoo and warm water. Two shampoos may be necessary. As mentioned, in step 4, if a large amount of oil was used, a mild liquid dish detergent will wash it out of the hair more quickly. *Do not use paint remover, paint thinner, turpentine, or cleaning fluid,* as these can burn the dog's skin.

7. To remove road tar, trim off as much tar-covered hair as possible. Rub butter, margarine, shortening, or vegetable oil into the remaining areas, and allow it to remain until the tar softens and can be removed. Wash with a mild liquid dishwashing detergent and warm water. Rinse well; repeat if necessary.

Inhaled Poisons

A dog can be poisoned by inhaling smoke, gas fumes, automobile exhaust (carbon monoxide), or chemical fumes from paints, refrigerants, solvents, or plastic and carbon compounds.

Symptoms of Inhaled Poisons

- Nausea.
- Sneezing.
- Dizziness.
- Breathing difficulties: rapid or slow respiration.
- Bright red color of mouth and tongue (carbon monoxide and cyanide exposure).
- Convulsions.
- Loss of consciousness.
- Shock.

Emergency Action for Inhaled Poisons

1. Move the dog away from the toxic environment into fresh air or a well-ventilated area.
2. Clear the air passages of accumulated material, if any. Remove the collar or anything tight around the neck that might obstruct breathing. Position the head to make breathing as free as possible.

3. If breathing has stopped, administer artificial respiration. (See "Artificial Respiration.")
4. Animals that inhale gases or toxic fumes suffer serious respiratory damage. Oxygen is of prime concern. *Remove the dog immediately to a veterinarian for oxygen and medical treatment.*
5. Treat for shock en route to veterinary hospital. (See "Shock.")

Injected Poisons

The bites of poisonous insects and snakes inject venom into the dog's body. For symptoms and emergency procedures, see "Insect bites and stings" and "Snakebite."

PORCUPINE QUILLS

Porcupines are found in many parts of the United States and Canada. They have stiff, sharp erectile quills of varying lengths covering most of their bodies (except feet, face, and underparts). A porcupine does not expel its quills, but when it is attacked they may detach and become embedded in the dog's muzzle or other parts of the body. Depending on the length of the dog-porcupine encounter, the dog can be stuck with quite a few quills. Removing the quills is a difficult, traumatic procedure. If there are many quills stuck in the skin, take the dog to a veterinarian as soon as possible to have them removed, as this painful procedure usually requires anesthesia.

Prevention

If you live in areas where there are porcupines, keep your dog from going into the woods or other overgrown areas, especially from dusk through the night—the time when the problem is most likely to occur.

Materials Required for Emergency Action

Long-nosed pliers or forceps

Emergency Action When a Veterinarian Is Not Available

1. Tie a safety muzzle around the dog's mouth (before doing this, see step 3). Try to restrain the dog when performing the following steps, although this may be difficult because it is in great pain. (See "Handling and Restraint.")
2. Use a pair of long-nosed pliers or a forceps. It is important to remove each *entire* quill, one by one. Grasp the quill near the point where it is embedded in the skin and pull it straight backward. Even though the dog may be fussy, try not to pull quills at an angle or they will break apart, leaving the lower parts stuck in the skin.
3. Do the muzzle and head first, as they usually get the most quills. Examine the inside of the mouth thoroughly *(don't muzzle the dog if there are quills in the tongue without first removing them)*. Then pull the quills from the rest of the body. There is a danger that deeply implanted quills or those that have broken apart cannot be removed and will move inward and cause infection or other problems.
4. Get to a veterinarian as soon as possible. Some deeply embedded quills may have to be removed surgically. Antibiotic treatment may be necessary.
5. For the next few days, examine the dog thoroughly to determine if any quills or broken parts are moving outward. Pull them out if you can.

Remember: Remove porcupine quills only when professional help is not immediately available.

RECTAL EMERGENCIES

Rectal emergencies are discussed at "Anal Gland Impaction," "Bloody Stools," "Constipation," "Diarrhea," "Foreign Objects, Swallowed or Embedded," and "Rectal Prolapse."

RECTAL PROLAPSE

In rectal prolapse, the lower part of the rectum and inside lining of the anus protude to look like a red hemorrhoid-size mass. Seen most often in puppies and older dogs, this condition can occur at any age. Severe diarrhea or straining from constipation are the principal causes of rectal prolapse.

Symptoms

- Licking and biting of protruding tissue.
- Swelling of protruding tissue.
- Discomfort and pain.

Materials Required for Emergency Action

Instant cold compress or ice
Germicidal soap

Emergency Action

1. Activate instant cold compress or place a small amount of crushed ice in a plastic bag. Wrap either in a towel and apply to the rectal area to reduce the swelling of protruding tissue.
2. Wash the area with germicidal soap and warm water to clean the exposed tissue. Rinse and dry thoroughly.
3. Wash your hands with germicidal soap and water and rinse well. Use one finger to gently replace the exposed tissue inside the rectum. If prolapse is difficult to replace, lubricate *slightly* with Vaseline®. (Over-lubrication often causes a recurrence of the condition.)
4. Remember that it will be necessary to treat the cause (diarrhea, constipation) to prevent further prolapsing.
5. Consult your veterinarian as soon as possible. Should there be additional prolapses, surgery may be necessary.

RESPIRATORY EMERGENCIES

(See "Artificial Respiration.")

SHOCK

Shock can be described as the partial or complete collapse of blood vessels that supply oxygen to the body's vital organs. In severe shock, the heart weakens; the blood flow is decreased and cannot meet the body's needs. *Time is critically important.* Without enough blood and oxygen, the vital organs—heart, kidneys, liver, brain—become depressed. If treatment is delayed, the depression cannot be reversed; the vital organs cease to function and the dog dies. Many deaths result from shock and not from what produced the shock.

Symptoms

Any or all of these may appear.
Early stages:

- Pale (often bluish or white) gums, inside of mouth, and eyelids.
- Weakness.
- Apathy.
- Cold and clammy feel to the skin.
- Rapid pulse rate which may be faint and difficult to detect.
- Rapid breathing which may be shallow or deep but irregular.
- Low body temperature. Rectal temperature often falls below 100°F.
- Vomiting.
- Diarrhea.

Advanced stages:*

---

* *These signs are ominous and indicate a serious condition; the dog is in danger of dying.*

- Eyes are indented and have a "glassy" expression.
- Pupils may be greatly enlarged.
- Collapse.
- Loss of consciousness.
- Coma.

PRIME OBJECTIVES IN TREATMENT OF SHOCK

1. To provide an open airway to receive sufficient oxygen.
2. To control or eliminate the cause of shock.
3. To restore efficient blood circulation.
4. To sustain normal body temperature.
5. To attend to other *serious* injuries.
6. To get professional help as soon as possible.

Materials Required for Emergency Action

Blanket
Dressings and bandage as necessary for injuries

Emergency Action

1. Provide an open airway to receive sufficient oxygen. Loosen the collar or anything tight around the dog's neck that obstructs breathing. Open the mouth, clean out mucus and foreign material, and pull the tongue forward.
2. Control or eliminate the cause of shock.
   a. If there is violent bleeding, control it immediately. (See "Bleeding.")
   b. If breathing is irregular or has stopped, give artificial respiration. (See "Artificial Respiration.")
   c. If the heart has stopped beating, give external heart massage. (See "Cardiac Arrest.")
3. Restore efficient blood circulation. The dog's best position is important: it depends on its injuries and the cause of shock. Generally it is most effective to place the dog on its side (if the surface is cold or damp, put a blanket down first) with the head even with or lower than the body level. *Do not reposition the body*

if severe head, neck, or spinal injuries are present; in this case, it is better to keep the dog lying flat. If the dog has severe chest injuries or is unconscious, it should be placed to allow effective drainage of fluids from the mouth to prevent choking.

4. Sustain normal body temperature.
   a. Keep the dog warm by covering it securely with a blanket.
   b. Do not overheat by adding heating appliances or hot packs, which can cause skin burns because of the system's poor circulation.
   c. Keep the dog as quiet as possible. Avoid noise that might encourage movement.
5. Attend to other *serious* injuries. Because it is important to reach a veterinarian as soon as possible, perform necessary first aid for serious emergencies only.
6. Go to a veterinarian immediately for administration of intravenous fluids and other medical treatment. Shock is a life-threatening emergency and, in advanced stages, quick action is necessary to save the dog's life.

If you cannot reach a veterinarian within the hour, liquids can be given by mouth. It is important to replace fluid loss, and often the dog will be thirsty. Give water or mix a solution of 1 level teaspoonful of salt and 1/2 level teaspoonful of baking soda in a quart of water. Depending on its size, allow the dog to sip 1 to 2 ounces of fluid every 15 minutes. Do not give liquids, however, if the dog:

1. Is unconscious.
2. Has convulsions.
3. Vomits or is liable to vomit.
4. Seems to have a severe brain, chest, or abdominal injury.
5. May need surgery because of extensive injuries.

Keep the dog warm and quiet until you can reach a veterinarian. Discontinue fluids if the dog becomes nauseated or begins to vomit.

SKULL FRACTURE

(See "Head Injuries.")

SKUNK ODOR

A dog that has been sprayed by a skunk needs immediate attention.

1. Even though the dog's smell is offensive, check the eyes first to determine if they have been sprayed, as skunk spray can be irritating to the eyes. Flush the eyes with lukewarm tap water under low pressure, holding the lids apart. Flushing should begin as soon as possible after irritation and continue for at least 5 minutes. After a thorough rinsing, apply a soothing eye ointment. (See recommendations in "Your Dog's First-Aid Kit.")
2. An effective way to neutralize skunk odor on the dog's body is to mix about 5 ounces of Massengill douche powder or liquid (available at most pharmacies) in 1 gallon of warm water. Saturate the hair with this mixture, taking care not to get it into the dog's eyes. *Do not rinse.* Allow the mixture to dry on the hair. Brush the hair as soon as it dries.
3. Other ways to neutralize skunk odor are:
   a. Place the dog in a tub and saturate the hair with tomato juice. On large breeds, several quarts of tomato juice may be necessary to soak the entire dog. Allow the juice to remain on the coat for about 15 minutes, then rinse it out. Follow the tomato juice treatment with a shampoo (two, if necessary) and a thorough rinsing.
   b. Rinse the dog with a mixture of clear ammonia and water (about 2 teaspoons ammonia per quart of water). Before rinsing the dog, coat the genitals with Vaseline®. Saturate the hair (do not get mixture into the eyes) and rinse as soon as possible. Be sure the ammonia mixture is rinsed thoroughly from the hair.

4. Depending on how badly the dog has been skunk-sprayed, it may be necessary to repeat your selected procedure several times.

SMOKE INHALATION

(See "Poisoning: Inhaled Poisons.")

SNAKEBITE

In every part of the world, more dogs than other domestic animals die from snakebite. This can be attributed to the small size of a dog in proportion to the degree of injected venom. Snakes most commonly bite dogs on the muzzle, shoulders, or legs. Any dog that is free to wander or exercise in areas known to harbor snakes can become a victim.

Nonpoisonous Snakes

Nonpoisonous snakes do not have fangs or true venom. The teeth leave fine U-shaped puncture marks (Illus. 46). The upper part of the head is covered with large scales and the eyes have round pupils. The wounds are usually not very painful but may swell slightly.

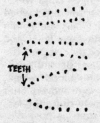

TEETH

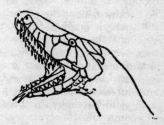

46. NONPOISONOUS SNAKE

Poisonous Snakes

Poisonous snakes have fangs through which they deliver their venom. For a dog to be poisoned, it must be punctured by one or more fangs. The bite leaves distinct punctures from fangs along the U-shaped marks from other teeth (Illus. 47).

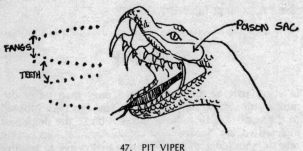

47. PIT VIPER

There are two types of venomous or poisonous snakes in North America: pit vipers, which include the American copperhead, the cotton-mouth (water moccasin), and all varieties of rattlesnakes; and the elapids, of which only coral snakes are found in the United States.

Pit vipers have a pit between the eye and nostril on each side of the head that operates as a specialized heat detector, enabling the snake to sense warm objects in front of it. The pits make these snakes very exact at judging distances; they can strike accurately at warm-blooded victims. Pit vipers have large hinged fangs which lie backward along the upper jaw and become erect when the snake is ready to strike. When pit vipers are within striking distance, they lunge swiftly with their fangs and then withdraw, seldom holding on to the victim. The venom breaks down the tissues and causes painful swellings and discolorations at the bite, injures blood vessels, and interferes with clotting. Even if a dog recovers after a pit viper bite, necrosis (tissue death) may cause the loss of a limb.

Elapine snakes have small fangs which are rigid in the upper jaw, erect and ready to strike. Elapine snakes hold on to and gnaw their prey. Their venom is highly neuro-toxic and may quickly produce convulsions, muscular weakness, shock, coma, or a paralysis that involves the muscles used in breathing, causing death by suffocation.

Symptoms of Bites from Poisonous Snakes

Any or all may be present.
Viperine snakes:

* Immediate swelling around bite. If a limb is bitten, its size may double.
* Intense burning and pain at bite.
* Discoloration of tissue at bite.
* Impaired vision.
* Nausea.
* Muscular weakness.
* Shock.

Elapine snakes: Bites produce little or no pain or swelling, but the following may develop rapidly:

* Muscular weakness.
* Convulsions.
* Respiratory paralysis.
* Shock.
* Coma.

Materials Required for Bites from Poisonous Snakes

Snakebite kit containing:

Instant cold compress
Tourniquet
Antiseptic wipes
Antiseptic
Sterile gauze dressings
Suction device
Scalpel or razor blade

	Appearance
American copperhead	Large crossbands of brown on pale salmon or reddish brown skin; copper tint on head. Grows to average length of $2^1/_2$–$3^1/_2$ feet.
Eastern diamondback rattlesnake[a]	Dark diamonds with lighter borders on a tan background. Dark bands on tail. Grows to average length of 5 feet.
Western diamondback rattlesnake[a]	Light brown to dark diamond shapes on tan, gray, or pinkish background. Black-and-white bands on tail. Grows to average of 4–5 feet long.
Timber rattlesnake[a]	Brown V-shaped patches on back on yellowish or ocher background. Grows to about 40 inches long.
Prairie rattlesnake[a]	Outlines of yellow or ocher diamonds on tan-pinkish background. Solid color head. Varies in length—not more than 5 feet long.
Pigmy rattlesnake[a]	Reddish and dark shapes down center of head and back on tan, olive, or brownish background. Shields on head. Grows 18–24 inches.

Territory	Remarks
In eastern United States from Florida to New England, found in wooded mountains, damp meadows, hills, often in woodsy suburbs; in south from Florida to Texas in uplands and lowland swamps	Of elusive disposition but may bite if irritatingly provoked. When irate, can vibrate its tail, sounding similar to a rattlesnake. Dreaded because of its fast strike.
In southeastern United States, south from North Carolina and west to Louisiana, often in thickets, palmettos, pines, or woods	Often lethargic, but may be dangerous since it may not rattle until directly approached. Usually will defend itself fiercely and not back away.
In southwestern states from Oklahoma to California in deserts and prairies; often near towns or farmland; sometimes along edges of mountain ranges or near coastal sand dunes	Very aggressive snake. Quick to rattle, coil, and strike when victim is in range. One of the main causes of snakebite and venom deaths in the United States.
In northeastern and central United States, mainly in rocky wooded country	Generally of peaceable disposition but will bite if cornered.
Found in prairies in western United States and southwestern Canada	Often moves about in daylight. In winter, goes below ground, often hibernating in prairie dog burrows.
Southeastern United States	Very quick-tempered. Since rattle is proportionately smaller, the sound is often heard only a short distance from snake.

	Appearance
Cottonmouth (water moccasin)	Dark blotches on olive or brown body. Broad and flat head. Heavy body. Grows to average of a little over 3 feet.
Coral snake	Bodies have bands of black, red and yellow rings. Average eastern species about 2 feet long. Arizona species about 20 inches long. Black nose.

Territory	Remarks
Mainly in swamps in southeastern United States, north to Virginia and west to Texas	Bite can be lethal. Lethargic and seldom moves when disturbed. When provoked, before biting it will open mouth wide to show white coloring inside. This is how snake got its name.
Eastern species found from Florida north to the Carolinas and west to Texas in dry woods and suburbs, often under logs, stones, or dense undergrowth; western species found in desert and semidesert of Arizona	In North American coral snakes, the red and yellow rings are always in contact. Certain harmless snakes are similarly colored, but there are black rings between any red or yellow bands. Coral snake venom is highly neurotoxic—respiratory paralysis and coma may occur quickly.

Source: Adapted from John Stidworthy, *Snakes of the World* (New York: Bantam Books.)

[a] Rattlesnakes comprise about 20 species, most of which are found in the United States. The singular feature that makes rattlesnakes different from other snakes is the development of the tail segments, which interlock. They are hollow and when moved, produce a noise called a rattle; however, the sound is not so much a rattle as a whirring noise. When a rattler is really provoked, the tail moves so fast that the sound becomes a buzz or blur.

Emergency Action for Bites from Poisonous Snakes

Speed is important to save the dog's life. Don't delay in reaching a veterinarian. The object of first aid for snakebite is to slow the spread of venom until a veterinarian can treat the dog with antivenin. Until help is obtained:

1. Place the dog at rest in a warm, quiet place. Avoid movement, exercise, or excitement, as this may help spread venom through the body.
2. If necessary, muzzle the dog before further treatment. (See "Handling and Restraint.")
3. Remove the hair from around the bite, if possible.
4. If the bite is on a limb, apply a moderately tight tourniquet about 2 inches above the wound. Do not tie the tourniquet so tightly that it stops the flow of blood into the leg; it should impede the blood flow in the veins, not the arteries. Leave the tourniquet in place for an hour or so. If the leg becomes very swollen, loosen the tourniquet slightly, but don't repeatedly release and reapply it.
5. Maintain the bitten part on a level with the heart to help prevent the spread of venom through the body.
6. Make two shallow lengthwise incisions through the skin using a razor blade, scalpel, or sharp knife. *Do not make crisscross incisions, as this may cause additional tissue damage.* Cut over the fang marks and over the suspected area of injected venom. Usually, snakes strike downward and the venom will be deposited just below the fang marks.
7. The incisions should not be more than 1/2 inch long. Be careful not to cut too deeply or you may sever muscles, nerves, tendons, veins, or arteries.
8. Remove venom and blood with a suction device. Do not withdraw the venom orally, if possible, especially if you have a cut or sore inside your mouth.
9. Apply antiseptic to the entire area.
10. Cover the wound with a sterile gauze dressing.
11. Place activated cold compress or ice wrapped in a towel immediately above the wound. Always wrap cold material in a towel, as freezing of the damaged tissues should be avoided.
12. Do not give any stimulant.

13. Watch for shock. (See "Shock.")
14. Check breathing often. If breathing stops, give artificial respiration. (See "Artificial Respiration.")
15. Consult a veterinarian at once where the dog will be given antivenin intravenously and additional medical treatment. If you have seen the snake that attacked your dog, try to remember as much as you can about it to help your veterinarian identify the correct species.

The seriousness of snake bite depends on the area of the wound and the type and amount of venom injected. Multiple bites are more serious since the snake injects some of its venom each time it strikes.

SPINAL INJURIES

Sudden fractures of the vertebral column (spine), ruptures of intervertebral disks or luxations (dislocations) can be caused by car accidents, heavy objects hitting the back, or severe falls or blows. A principal function of the spine is to protect the spinal cord contained within it. Once the spine is fractured or vertebra dislocated, the spinal cord is in danger at the injury point. If you feel that your dog may have a spinal injury, careful handling is very important.

In addition, dogs can develop tumors, disk degeneration, or other conditions which result in progressive spinal cord damage. These may be only slightly painful at first, with recurrent attacks that become more serious. Eventually, the slightest overexertion will cause a worsening of the condition. In a progressive condition, treatment may involve the use of drugs for pain, muscle relaxants, corticosteroids, or surgery.

Symptoms (Depending on Injury)

- Staggering gait.
- Extreme pain.
- Breathing difficulties (injuries of the neck vertebrae).
- Rigidity of legs.

177

- Tenseness of abdomen.
- Partial paralysis of hind or front legs.
- Little or no pain response. Loss of feeling on front or hind legs when pinched.
- Loss of bladder or bowel function.
- Total paralysis.
- Shock.

Emergency Action

1. Careful handling is important. Do not bend, twist, or move the dog's body unless it is absolutely necessary.
2. If breathing is difficult, make sure airways are open and free of obstruction. Head movement should be minimal: *do not move from side to side, forward, or backward.*
3. If breathing has stopped, give artificial respiration. (See "Artificial Respiration.")
4. Remove the dog at once to a veterinarian. Extreme care must be taken, when you move a spine-injured dog, to keep the head and body as rigid as possible. Try to have at least one other person help you move the dog.
5. Patients should be moved on a carrying device. *Do not twist or bend the dog's body when slipping support underneath*. Use the following steps to transfer the dog onto a carrying device (see Illus. 2, 3):
   a. Large breeds: As the dog lies on its side, place a board, table pad, etc., of sufficient width parallel to the dog, under both sets of legs. Grasp the front and back legs and gently and evenly pull the dog, legs first, until the body is squarely centered on the board.
   b. Medium and small breeds: Place a board, table pad, etc., of sufficient width parallel to the dog's spine. Grasp the skin at the back of the neck and on the back and gently and evenly slip the dog, body first, onto the board until it is squarely centered. If you do not have a board or table pad, use a cardboard box with one side removed.

   A blanket can be used as a carrying device; it *must* be placed on something rigid before being lifted to support the dog's body.

6. Place rolled-up towels around the body for support. If necessary, secure the dog to the board with bandage, straps, or other type of tie to immobilize the spine during travel.
7. Load and unload the car with great caution. Avoid unnecessary movement or jarring of the body.
8. Treat for shock, if necessary. (See "Shock.")

Note: Illustrations for these instructions and additional information for moving seriously injured dogs can be found in "Emergency Transportation of Injured Dogs."

SUFFOCATION OR ASPHYXIA

(See "Artificial Respiration.")

URINARY TRACT EMERGENCIES

Urinary tract conditions requiring emergency treatment are ruptured bladder, cystitis, and obstructions/stones.

Ruptured Bladder

A rupture of the bladder may occur if a dog is hit by an automobile, suffers a fall, is kicked, or receives some other kind of severe blow.

Symptoms of Ruptured Bladder

- Difficulty in passing urine.
- Absence of urination.
- Abdominal pain.
- Blood in urine.
- Distended abdomen.
- Collapse.
- Shock.

Emergency Action for Ruptured Bladder

1. Consult your veterinarian immediately, as this is a serious condition which requires surgery.

Cystitis

Cystitis or inflammation of the bladder can be caused by bacterial infections, bladder tumors, or diet (occasionally), but most of the time the condition is associated with urinary calculi (stones).

Symptoms of Cystitis

* Frequent squatting and straining to urinate.
* Increased urination.
* Blood in urine.
* Ammonia-smelling urine.
* Abdominal pain.
* Elevated temperature (not always present).
* Excessive licking of the vulva (female).

Emergency Action for Cystitis

1. Consult a veterinarian immediately. Treatment varies depending on the cause. Bacterial infections are treated with antibiotics. X rays may be required if the veterinarian believes the condition is caused by something other than infection.
2. If possible, take along a fresh urine sample for analysis.

Urinary Tract Obstructions/Stones

Urinary tract obstructions or stones may form in the dog's bladder, ureter, urethra, or kidney. Stones vary in size; depending on their location, they can cause great pain and partial or complete obstruction of urine. In dogs, males have more problems than females because of differences in anatomy. The male's discharge passage (urethra) is narrow and restricted by the os penis or bony structure which surrounds it and can become obstructed easily with stones. The female's urethra is wider and not as easily obstructed; some small stones can be passed without causing much pain. At a dog health seminar sponsored by the Morris Animal Foundation of Denver, Dr. Michael Lorenz said that "most stones are classified by their mineral composition. If you have a dog with bladder stones or stones in the urinary system which are removed, it is very important to have them analyzed, and it is well worth the expense. Definitive treatment of this condition can be made after it is known what kind of stone is located in the urinary tract. The most common type of stones in the urinary tracts of dogs are phosphate stones, or triple phosphate calculi. Of all uroliths (stones in the urinary tract) 69% are composed of phosphate. These stones occur in many breeds, including mongrels. But in general the chondrodystroid breeds (like Bulldogs and Dachshunds, which have short extremities or noses) are predisposed to urinary calculi of all types."

Symptoms of Urinary Tract Obstructions/Stones

- Frequent squatting and straining to urinate.
- Frequent passing of small amounts of urine.
- Complete absence of urine.
- Blood in urine.
- Extreme pain (back or abdomen).
- Thirst.

Emergency Action for Urinary Tract Obstructions/Stones

1. Consult a veterinarian immediately, as this is a serious condition which needs immediate relief. Treatment varies depending on the type and location of stones. Treatment usually involves surgery.

UTERINE INFECTIONS

Pyrometra

Pyrometra is a uterine infection that is seen most often in unspayed females over 5 years old. It occurs after the heat cycle and is believed to be the result of hormone disturbance. If the cervix remains open, there is a smelly, reddish purulent discharge from the vulva; if the cervix closes, the uterus becomes enlarged and fills with pus.

Either type of pyrometra is serious and requires immediate veterinary treatment.

Symptoms of Pyrometra

- Reddish mucus discharge (not always present).
- Listlessness.
- Lack of appetite.
- Increased thirst.
- Vomiting.
- Increased urination.
- Abdominal swelling.
- Fever (not always present).

Emergency Action for Pyrometra

Take the dog to the veterinarian for immediate treatment. If pyrometra is ignored, the results can be fatal.

Metritis

Metritis is an inflammation of the uterus that occurs after whelping. (See "Postwhelping Complications: Metritis" in section III.)

VOMITING

Vomiting is a reflex action in which the stomach's contents are forcibly ejected through the mouth. Dogs can initiate this reflex action quickly and easily as a protective measure to rid the stomach of grass, spoiled food, garbage, or other irritating materials. Nervous dogs often vomit because of changes in diet, excitement, or overactivity. If your dog vomits for a short time from these causes, without temperature rise or abdominal pain, the vomiting usually can be handled by home treatment.

However, persistent vomiting (often containing blood, bile, or excessive mucus) is a symptom of many illnesses, including intestinal parasites, distemper, hepatitis, intestinal obstructions, poisoning, pancreatitis, peritonitis, tumor, ulcers, and kidney problems. Consult a veterinarian as soon as possible, for without prompt medical treatment persistent vomiting will dehydrate and further debilitate a sick pet.

It is important to know the difference between vomiting, as defined above, and regurgitation, which is the ejection of undigested food from the mouth or esophagus. Food is regurgitated while or shortly after eating and appears to be compressed into a sausage shape. Frequent regurgitation is a symptom of esophagus or pharynx problems and requires veterinary attention as soon as possible.

Symptoms

- Restlessness.
- Salivation.
- Frequent swallowing.
- Licking of lips.
- Intermittent contractions of the abdomen.

Action for Vomiting of Short Duration

1. Withhold food and water for 12 to 24 hours to rest the stomach. Otherwise, further irritation of the stomach may cause more vomiting.
2. Give small quantities (a few teaspoons every hour) of liquid that has been boiled, then cooled to room temperature, bottled water, soda water, 7-Up, or Gatorade if they can be retained. If not and the dog is thirsty, let it lick ice cubes frequently.
3. To help soothe stomach irritation, give any antacid product with a protective coating action, such as Pepto-Bismol®, Maalox®, Kaopectate, or Mylanta®. Give 1 to 2 teaspoons per 20 pounds of body weight every 4 to 6 hours until symptoms have passed.
4. Keep the dog warm and quiet. Restrict activity; allow the pet to rest as much as possible.
5. When vomiting stops, begin feeding small meals consisting of bland food: boiled rice, chicken or beef broth, baby cereals, cooked egg, boiled *lean* chopped beef or lamb. Avoid fatty foods.
6. As the dog improves, feed regular-size portions of bland food the next day, then return to normal diet.

Action for Vomiting of Long Duration

If the vomiting persists longer than 24 hours, consult your veterinarian as soon as possible. Vomiting can be a sign of a number of serious illnesses.

WOUNDS, CLOSED

A closed wound or contusion is an injury in which there is no break in the skin. The tissues beneath the skin may have been injured by a blow from a blunt object, an automobile accident, or jumping or falling from high places. Such injuries can occur in any area of the dog's body. The danger of infection is not great, since closed wounds are subject to little contamination. A closed wound may be a minor injury—a bruise, for example—which damages the soft tissues beneath the skin; or it may be serious and cause considerable internal bleeding (see "Bleeding: Internal Bleeding") and extensive damage to deeper tissues and organs.

Symptoms

These depend on the type of object striking the blow and the location involved.

* Restlessness.
* Pain and tenderness in area of suspected injury.
* Swelling.
* Discoloration from rupturing of capillaries in affected area.
* Cold and clammy feel to the skin.
* Excessive thirst.
* Distortion of a leg as a result of a fracture or dislocation.
* Rapid and weak pulse.
* Rapid and shallow breathing.
* Blood vomited or present in urine or bowel movements.
* Staggering gait.
* Loss of consciousness.
* Coma.
* Shock.

Materials Required for Emergency Action

Cold compresses or ice
Blanket
Firm object for transportation (for deep closed wounds)

Emergency Action for Superficial Contusions

1. If the injury is relatively minor, apply a cold compress or ice pack to the area of the bruise to help prevent swelling and to lessen internal bleeding. Cold compresses should be applied to the bruised part as soon as possible after the injury and kept in place for about 15 to 20 minutes. Repeat every 2 hours.
2. Keep the dog quiet. Do not allow exercise or activity that will aggravate the injury.

Emergency Action for Deep Closed Wounds

1. Assure a clear airway. Loosen the collar or anything tight around the dog's neck that might obstruct breathing.
2. Place the dog in a comfortable position and inspect the body for fractures, dislocations, and other injuries to the head, neck, back, chest, abdomen, or legs:
   a. If a fracture, dislocation, or sprain is suspected, splint or immobilize the injured part before moving the dog. (See "Fractures, Dislocations, Sprains, and Strains.")
   b. If an internal injury or bleeding is suspected, seek veterinary help immediately. (See "Bleeding: Internal Bleeding.")
   c. In either case, the body should be kept in a prone position and moved carefully. Step-by-step directions for moving seriously injured dogs are found in "Emergency Transportation of Injured Dogs."
   d. Do not give anything by mouth if you suspect an internal injury.
   e. Keep the dog warm by wrapping with a blanket. Treat for shock if necessary. (See "Shock.")
   f. Get the dog to a veterinarian immediately.

WOUNDS, OPEN

An open wound is a break in the dog's skin. Because there is a danger of bleeding and contamination, first aid for open wounds should consist of controlling bleeding and preventing infection. Types of open wounds include:

1. Abrasions or scrapes: Wounds made by rubbing or scraping against a hard surface and causing damage to the skin's outer layers. Usually, bleeding is superficial because the wound is not deep.
2. Cuts or incisions: Wounds made by sharp or cutting objects such as broken glass, rough metal edges, and knives. The amount of bleeding depends on the extent of damage but can be profuse. Deep incisions can sever veins and arteries and injure muscles and tendons and other tissues.
3. Lacerations: Wounds that result in jagged breaks or tears in the skin. These are usually caused by animal bites, barbed wire, or blunt objects. Tissue damage from a laceration is more extensive than from a cut; since a laceration can penetrate deeply into the tissues, there is a danger of profuse bleeding.
4. Punctures: Wounds that result in small openings in the skin from sharp-pointed or penetrating objects like pins, nails, thorns, bullets, fishhooks, and cat bites. Punctures may appear small on the skin surface but can penetrate deeply into the tissues and cause serious damage. External bleeding may be limited because the wound can close quickly; but there may be internal bleeding and infection with an abscess developing.
5. Avulsions: Wounds that cause the tissue to be torn or separated violently from the body, as a result of an automobile or other serious accident, explosions, gunshots, animal bites, etc. There may be instant and massive bleeding.

Wounds with Massive Bleeding

Emergency procedures for wounds with massive bleeding will be found at "Bleeding."

Symptoms of Minor Wounds

- Pain.
- Swelling and tenderness of specific area.
- Hair loss.
- Constant licking.
- Blood matted on coat.
- Opening in the skin.

Materials Required for Minor Wounds

Germicidal soap
Sterile gauze dressings
Bandage
Blunt-tipped scissors
Adhesive tape
Antiseptic skin ointment

Emergency Action for Minor Wounds

1. Muzzle or restrain the dog if necessary. (See "Handling and Restraint.")
2. Wash your hands thoroughly with soap and water.
3. Clip the hair from the area around the wound with blunt-tipped scissors.
4. Clean the wound with tincture of green soap or other germicidal soap and water. Rinse thoroughly.
5. Blot dry with a sterile gauze dressing if available.
6. Use a moistened cotton swab or the corner of a sterile gauze dressing and carefully remove any hair or foreign matter from the wound.
7. Apply an antiseptic or antiseptic skin ointment.
8. Cover the wound with a sterile gauze dressing. (See "Bandaging.") If necessary, apply additional dressings for padding before bandaging the wound.
9. Bandage and tape the dressings in place. (See "Bandaging.")
10. Redress the wound every second day. Check for signs of infection. (If the wound becomes infected, see "Wounds, Open: Infected Wounds" and consult your veterinarian as soon as possible.)

Dogs Bitten by Animals

Dogs are often bitten by other dogs or cats. The severity of the bite depends on the location of the wound, whether it is a tear or a puncture, and the size of the animal that did the biting.

Animal bites can be painful and potentially dangerous if the wound is a deep puncture. When an animal's tooth penetrates the dog's skin, it can cause external tissue damage and also internal damage to muscles and blood vessels that may not be readily apparent.

Cat bites can be serious too. They may look like insignificant punctures and heal quickly on the skin surface, but because the wound is unable to drain, an abscess can form underneath. Bite wounds must be allowed to drain freely and should be kept open and permitted to heal from the inside out. Any deep puncture is likely to become infected and should be treated by a veterinarian.

Materials Required for Dogs Bitten by Animals

Germicidal soap
Hydrogen peroxide
Sterile gauze dressings
Bandage
Adhesive tape
Antiseptic skin ointment or antiseptic such as tincture of
  Merthiolate

Emergency Action for Dogs Bitten by Animals

1. Muzzle and restrain the dog if necessary. (See "Handling and Restraint.")
2. Wash your hands thoroughly with soap and water.
3. Wash the wound with germicidal soap and water. If the injury is a deep puncture, flush out the area with a 3% solution of Hydrogen Peroxide to remove bacteria or other foreign matter.
4. Blot the wound with a sterile gauze dressing if available.
5. Apply antiseptic or antiseptic skin ointment.
6. Dress and bandage the wound. (See "Bandaging.")

7. Flush and redress the wound every day. Check for the presence of infection. (See "Wounds, Open: Infected Wounds.")
8. Large wounds usually will require sutures. Take the dog to a veterinarian as soon as possible.

Humans Bitten by Animals

When a pet or wild animal bites a human, punctures, lacerations, or avulsions can be caused. Animal bites can be painful and potentially dangerous if the wound is deep. When animal teeth penetrate the skin, they can cause external tissue damage and internal damage to muscles and blood vessels that may not be readily apparent.

Humans are most often bitten by dogs and cats. A dog bite may cause more tissue damage (depending on the dog's size) than a cat bite; but cat bites can be just as hazardous, due to the greater number of bacteria in the mouth of a cat.

The threat of infection and the danger of tetanus and rabies are present in every animal bite. Besides dogs and cats, wild animals such as skunks, foxes, bats, raccoons, wolves, and coyotes transmit rabies, an infection whose virus is found in an infected animal's saliva. Once bitten, if the rabies virus is transmitted to a person, it goes through an incubation period that varies in duration. (See "Immunization Against Infectious Diseases: Rabies" in section IV.)

Anyone who is bitten by an animal *not positively* known to him or her should proceed as follows:

1. While most animals are not rabid, it is important that the biting animal be confined or captured and kept under observation for a required period of time to see if it develops the final stages of rabies.
2. Try to restrain or contain the animal or secure positive identification to locate its owner. Make every effort not to allow the animal to escape, but don't risk additional bites! If the animal does run away, follow it if you can, or determine the direction in which it escapes. Remember as much about the animal's appearance as you can (particularly if it is wear-

ing a collar or license). Ask neighbors or anyone in the area if they can identify the animal.
3. If the animal can be restrained, call your local ASPCA or Humane Society for help in capturing it.
4. Check with the police, veterinarian, or public health officials: the animal may have to be quarantined for observation.
5. Notify your physician immediately after any bite, regardless of whether the animal can be captured. Your physician may give a tetanus injection, tetanus toxoid booster, and possibly antibiotics.

Emergency Action for Humans Bitten by Animals

1. Clean the wound carefully with antibacterial soap, then flush with plenty of warm water.
2. Blot the area dry with a sterile dressing. Do not use antiseptics or other medications on a bite wound.
3. Apply a sterile dressing or clean cloth over the wound. Secure in place with bandage.
4. If the biting animal is suspected to be rabid, avoid moving your arms and legs until medical treatment is received.
5. Notify your physician as soon as possible after any animal bite.

Infected Wounds

The danger of infection is present in all open wounds. Even if the wound is minor and steps are taken to avoid contamination, bacteria can enter an open wound and infection can develop. Infected wounds should receive veterinary treatment as soon as possible.

Symptoms of Infected Wounds

- Pain.
- Swelling, redness, and tenderness of affected area.
- Elevated temperature.
- Wound feels hot to the touch.
- Presence of pus, either draining from the wound or encrusted around the wound or on the dressing.

Materials Required for Infected Wounds

Saline solution (make at home by mixing 1 level teaspoon
    of salt with 1 pint of hot—but not boiling—water)
Antiseptic skin ointment
Sterile gauze dressings
Bandage
Adhesive tape

Emergency Action for Infected Wounds

1. Keep the dog quiet. Do not allow exercise or activity that will aggravate the infection.
2. Carefully remove the bandages from the infected area.
3. Make a saline solution by mixing 1 teaspoon of salt with 1 pint of hot water.
4. Soak a towel or washcloth in the saline solution, wring it out, and place it over the wound for 15 to 20 minutes.
5. Repeat the heat applications for 15 to 20 minutes every hour.
6. Irrigate the wound thoroughly with the saline solution to clear away any purulent matter.
7. Blot dry with a sterile dressing.
8. Apply antiseptic skin ointment.
9. Cover with a clean sterile gauze dressing. Bandage and tape the dressing in place. (See "Bandaging.")
10. Consult a veterinarian as soon as possible.

Remember: These instructions are for temporary treatment only. Don't postpone seeing a veterinarian.

HOME NURSING: CONVALESCENT CARE OF SICK, INJURED, AND POSTOPERATIVE DOGS

There are few dogs that do not experience at least one illness which requires nursing care during convalescence. Whether a dog is sick, injured, or recuperating from an operation, the love, moral support, and competent care you give play an important part in recovery.

Many illnesses and injuries do not require hospitalization, but may require long periods of convalescence. How quickly the dog recovers can depend on the quality and consistency of care it receives. Even when hospitalization is neccessary, more and more veterinarians believe in releasing a dog as soon as possible after treatment or surgery for care at home, because most animals recover faster in familiar surroundings. When a dog, especially a pet, is in strange surroundings, it can grieve for its loved ones and become despondent, leading to loss of appetite and a progressive depression which can delay the healing process.

When you accept the responsibility of caring for a sick or postoperative dog at home, your veterinarian will usually provide specific instructions. These should be followed as closely as possible. Home nursing does not require much technical skill, but it does call for a combination of consistency, observation, common sense, and tenderness. How closely you follow the veterinarian's instructions will often determine how effective treatment will be. If you provide the basics, your dog's chances for recovery will be increased.

You should know how to take temperature, check pulse, observe changes in respiration, give medicines, and apply dressings and bandages. You must also make a commitment to follow special dietary instructions when necessary, to provide the correct atmosphere for convalescence, to keep the dog clean, and to observe changes in condition.

If you feel you cannot provide these basics or carry out the veterinarian's orders because your time is occupied with the care of small children or a job, then perhaps the dog should remain in the hospital for professional care. Nursing sick dogs is much like nursing sick children —it is time consuming and demands cheerfulness and patience. As a rule, dogs make excellent patients, especially when they are happy in their surroundings and have confidence in their nurse. Usually they will submit without protest even when unpleasant procedures must be carried out; often they show their gratitude in a poignant manner.

SELECTING THE CONVALESCENT AREA

A sick or invalid dog needs a special place in which to recuperate; this area should be selected and prepared in advance. Consider your dog's personality and temperament. Is the dog outgoing or nervous? Is total peace and quiet necessary? Are there small children or other pets in the house?

Depending on your dog's physical and mental condition, the recovery area can be a corner in the kitchen, den, or living room where the dog can be near the family, or a separate room away from the noise and commotion of family life.

Unless the pet is seriously ill or has something contagious—conditions which necessitate isolation—complete separation from others is not necessary so long as the convalescent area is in a quiet location. Whatever area is selected, the dog must be able to have total rest and quiet with as little excitement and handling as possible. Well-meaning but enthusiastic children or other pets in the family should not be permitted to disturb the patient. If isolation is necessary, be sure to look in on the dog frequently; when you do, stroke the dog gently and offer words of encouragement. A dog's sickroom should not be allowed to become its prison. When an invalid dog is left alone in a remote section of the house without regular contact, it feels cut off from the world. Take every opportunity to let your dog know you care. Arrange to write letters, read, mend clothes, or do needlework or other noiseless activities in the patient's room. Your presence will have a comforting effect.

The convalescent area should be warm and well ventilated, but not drafty. If the area is too bright, you should be able to draw the drapes or blinds if necessary: many illnesses make a dog's eyes extra-sensitive to light. The sickroom, however, must not be totally dark and depressing.

The temperature of the convalescent area should be between 60°F and 70°F (16°C to 21°C) depending on the environment the dog has been accustomed to. A dog that has lived outdoors most of its life will be comfortable with an inside temperature of 60°F (16°C), while an indoor dog will be more comfortable at 70°F (21°C). Remember that hot air rises and cool air falls; while you may be perfectly comfortable in the room, your dog may be chilled. If you are in doubt about the floor temperature, measure with a thermometer close to where the dog will be resting.

Whether the dog can go outside to urinate or have a bowel movement depends on the severity of the illness and time of year. When possible, a house-trained dog should be taken outside, as it can become very disturbed if it has to relieve itself indoors. Attach the lead and collar (and wear a coat in cold weather) and take the dog out to prevent overexercising. If the dog is unable to go outside because it is seriously ill or the weather is bad, relief may be a problem. It may be necessary to remove the carpets from the convalescent area, or if this is not possible, to spread a large plastic shower curtain, liner, or tablecloth on top of the carpet and cover it with newspapers.

The Bed

Provide a comfortable bed for the dog and place it in a warm, draft-free area. The bed should be large enough for the dog to stretch or turn with ease. Line the bed with freshly laundered sheets, towels, and a blanket or other soft material that can be cleaned easily. Keep the area clean and change the bedding regularly. Do remember that an invalid dog may not be able to control its elimination; if an accident occurs in the bed, change the bedding material as soon as possible.

Supplying the Sickroom

Once you have selected and prepared the convalescent area, add the materials and supplies the patient will require. You can keep a fresh change of bedding, clean towels, dressings and bandage (if necessary), cotton balls or swabs, a washcloth and plastic dishpan (for cleaning the dog), a brush or comb, scissors, grooming or talcum powder, a notebook and pen) and all necessary ointments and medications on a small table near the dog's bed. Of course, if you have small children or other pets in the family, you will want to keep all drugs in a safe place to avoid accidental poisoning.

The table should be the equivalent of a hospital cart; how it is stocked depends on the dog's illness and the length of time estimated for the healing process.

CARE OF THE CONVALESCENT DOG

Grooming

Grooming is an important part of nursing. A dog that is recovering from an illness or operation should be groomed every other day if it is well enough. Gentle brushing or combing helps clean the skin and makes the dog less susceptible to skin disease and parasites. Brushing helps distribute the hair's natural oils and, on long-coated breeds, removes the dead hair before it has a chance to mat. If the dog cannot move from its bed, try to lightly brush the hair with a soft bristle brush or to massage the skin and hair with your fingertips. This will not only make your dog look better but make it more comfortable.

Keeping the Dog Clean

Even if a bath is out of the question, a sick dog should be kept scrupulously clean. Sponging (not overwetting) the face and body is refreshing at any time of the year, especially in hot weather. Sponge baths can help reduce an elevated temperature. If vomiting or diarrhea occurs, the dog should be spot-cleaned soon after it becomes soiled.

Moisten a washcloth or small hand towel with warm water and a little mild shampoo, then gently sponge the face and body or spot-clean any soiled parts. Rinse with dampened washcloths dipped in clear water. Dry the area thoroughly and sprinkle with a little grooming or talcum powder.

The nose and eyes should be cleaned if there is a discharge in either area. Moisten a washcloth in warm water and gently wipe over the face. If any matter has accumulated and caked in the eye corners or around the nostrils, soften it first with warm water, then remove the accumulation with a cotton ball or Q-Tip. If the eyes are inflamed or have a heavy discharge, ask your veterinarian about the use of an ophthalmic ointment. When a respiratory ailment causes a mucous discharge, a vaporizer may help to keep the chest and nose free of congestion. After eating or periods of vomiting, clean the inside of the mouth, the gums, and teeth by wiping with a damp cloth.

Other aspects of cleanliness depend on how sick the dog is. If it can move around, the dog can relieve itself on newspaper that is provided in the recovery area. If the dog cannot walk, then *expect urination and bowel movements to occur in the bed.* Place a layer of plastic or rubber sheeting in the bottom of the bed, then line the bed with soft material that can be laundered easily, as the bedding may have to be changed frequently. Disposable baby diapers or disposable underpads (a special type made for dogs is available at most pet shops) can be arranged under the hindquarters to help keep the pet clean.

When the bedding is changed after an "accident," remember to sponge off the hindquarters and legs with a damp cloth to keep urine or feces from irritating the skin. After diarrhea, the dog should be washed as soon as it becomes soiled, for traces of stool that remain on the hair can harden and be difficult to remove and, on coated breeds, can form a seal over the rectum. A mild antiseptic ointment should be used on the anal area if it becomes inflamed. For coated breeds it is often easier to keep the dog clean by temporarily shortening the hair under the tail, below the rectum, and on the back legs.

Exercise

The person in charge of the recuperating dog should learn

from the veterinarian if mild exercise is permitted or if the dog should be kept as quiet as possible. Most dogs do not have to remain inactive for long periods after an illness or operation unless they are so weak or debilitated that complete rest and quiet are required—and when this is true, the dog will usually have to remain in the hospital.

Unless your veterinarian advises otherwise, mild exercise is usually beneficial while the dog is recovering. A sick dog should not be permitted to go outdoors in very cold or wet weather, but a brief period of fresh air and mild weather will be healthful to most convalescing dogs, even if the pet has to be carried outside and held in your arms for a few minutes. Restrict exercise at first, but as the dog begins to recover, gradually resume normal indoor, then outdoor activities.

Sickroom Procedures

When you are nursing a sick dog, remember that quiet, rest, gentle handling, love, and observation are essential for recovery. The dog should be handled gently and calmly and given a great deal of love and encouragement. Always maintain a cheerful attitude when you are attending to the dog, even if you are not in the best of moods, since dogs are very sensitive to voice intonations.

A patient that is very sick or weak needs special attention because it may not be able to accomplish things on its own. For instance, the dog may not be able to move toward its food or water dish or turn over in bed. You may have to support or hold the food or water bowl close to the patient instead of just sitting it in the bed next to the dog. If the dog is paralyzed or so weak that movement is not possible, it should be turned from side to side several times a day (every 2 to 3 hours) to prevent bedsores from forming. Bedsores are large, irritated areas which are caused by pressure. They are difficult to cure: if bedsores appear, notify your veterinarian at once. Bedsores can be prevented by providing soft and comfortable bedding, by changing the bedding regularly, by keeping the dog clean, and by turning it carefully and frequently.

Keep a notebook and pen in the sickroom to record

daily observations on the dog's recovery. If you accept the responsibility of nursing a dog that is recovering from an injury, illness, or operation, results are better when the "nurse" and veterinarian keep each other fully informed throughout the healing period. There are several visual and manual inspections you can make to determine if your dog is recovering; these should be recorded carefully in your notebook so that when you give the veterinarian a report, he will receive accurate facts. Remember, even though your dog cannot describe its problems or pains in words, you can usually determine potentially dangerous situations from the dog's actions and appearance.

Information recorded should include:

1. The date.

2. The dog's temperature. This should be measured rectally every morning and evening.

3. Breathing: Is respiration normal, rapid, shallow, or strained?

4. Pulse: Is the pulse normal, rapid, or weak?

5. Bowel movements: How often did the dog have a bowel movement? What was the consistency of each movement—normal, loose, hard, or bloody?

6. Urination: Is urination frequent or infrequent? Is there a normal or unusual color or odor?

7. Eyes: Are the eyes clear or cloudy? Is there a discharge? Are the eyes sensitive to light?

8. Nose: Is there a discharge?

9. Eating and drinking: Is the appetite normal? Is the dog eating less or refusing to eat? Are there changes in drinking habits?

10. Is the dog nauseated or vomiting? Does this happen after eating, or after medication?

11. Medication: Are you following the veterinarian's prescribed dosage schedule as closely as possible? If not, why not?

12. Movement: Is the dog walking normally? Is it unable to move? Is there any stiffness of the hindquarters or staggering gait?

13. General condition: Is the dog alert and interested? Is it drowsy and uninterested? Are there signs of pain or restlessness?

Depending on the nature of the illness, there may be other unusual signs you will notice: these should be recorded and reported to your veterinarian when you give a progress check. *Any dramatic changes in a sick dog's condition should be reported at once.*

Feeding a Sick Dog

The nutritional needs of a sick dog may differ from those of a healthy dog, depending on the type and severity of the illness, the dog's general condition, and the nutrients required for recovery.

Usually your veterinarian will prescribe the proper diet when your dog is recovering from a serious illness. Once an accurate diagnosis of the illness is made, your veterinarian will determine if modifications to the diet are necessary. Selecting the proper food for a sick dog requires as much knowledge as prescribing the correct medicine to treat a disease.

Often a Prescription Diet® will be recommended. This includes special formulas for postoperative cases, kidney ailments, congestive heart failure, intestinal problems, food-induced allergies, obesity, and other conditions. If your veterinarian suggests a Prescription Diet® or a home-prepared controlled diet, follow the instructions as closely as possible and *don't feed anything else.* Add vitamin supplements only if they are prescribed. Supplementation is necessary only when nutrients are lacking.

If you receive no special feeding instructions, try to make the regular diet more appetizing by adding a little beef or chicken broth to the food. Many convalescing dogs will refuse to eat their normal food; if this happens, you may have to experiment with different combinations of food until you determine what will stimulate the appetite. A mixture of cooked rice and ground beef or chicken often works well.

If your dog cannot keep its food down, try giving meals of nourishing bland foods that are easy to digest, such as cottage cheese, beef broth, and boiled eggs. Instead of feeding a large amount at one time, give the dog four or five small meals. Then as the dog improves, gradually increase the amounts until normal portions and food can be resumed. Consult your veterinarian if vomiting persists.

A dog that is convalescing must eat whether it wants to or not. When a dog refuses to eat (anorexia), it will begin to lose weight. Because no nutrients are being taken in, an anorectic dog uses its own body to obtain the nourishment necessary for life functions. When extra demands from disease are present, the deterioration is even faster. Steps to restore the food intake should begin immediately with or without the dog's consent. Often force feeding will be necessary.

Liquid foods can be given like liquid medicine. (See "How to Give Medicine: Giving Liquids by the Lip-Pocket Method.") The implement used to force-feed the liquid can be a spoon, feeding cup, kitchen poultry baster, or syringe (without the needle attached).

Hospital Diet® starter (available from veterinarians) or the following diet* meets all the normal fluid, electrolyte, and nutrient requirements of dogs and cats. Mix in a blender:

> 20 ounces water
> 8 ounces Prescription Diet® i/d®
> 2 ounces corn oil

The mixture should be stored in the refrigerator and warmed to body temperature prior to administration. It should be fed at the rate of 1 ounce per pound of body weight per day. If the animal has not been eating for more than 2 days, divide the initial daily dose into two or three feedings. Supply additional water to replace abnormal losses, such as those resulting from diarrhea or vomiting.

When force-feeding liquids, give small quantities at a time to prevent choking. After the dog has finished eating, if there is spilled liquid on the coat, wipe it clean with a damp cloth.

Solid foods like Prescription Diet,® cooked egg, baby foods, cereals, cottage cheese, and chopped meats can be force-fed. However, before resorting to forcing solids, try to tempt the dog to eat the food naturally. Smear a little of the food on the dog's teeth; put some food on the fingertips and let the dog lick it off, or offer a small amount of food in the palm of your hand. There is nothing

---

* Diet supplied by Dr. Mark L. Morris, Jr.

wrong with hand feeding a sick dog if this is the only way it will take food.

When force-feeding solid food, it can be compressed into small balls, which are placed (one at a time) in the mouth on the back of the tongue, in the same manner as you give a pill or capsule. (See "How to Give Medicines: Giving Pills or Capsules.")

Another method of force-feeding solid food, such as a Prescription Diet® or other food from a can, is to use a small disposable syringe, after using a sharp knife to cut off the end where the needle is normally attached. Be sure to smooth away any rough edges, to prevent the dog's mouth from being cut. Push the open end of the syringe into the food. As you do this, the plunger will rise as the barrel is being filled. Carefully twist the syringe out of the can, place it into the dog's mouth, depress the plunger and eject the core of food into the dog's mouth.

When you are force-feeding solids, don't force large quantities of food into the mouth at one time and don't become impatient if the dog resists. Stroke the dog, speak lovingly and reassuringly, and when things quiet down, try again. Force feeding requires a lot of patience and understanding.

If the dog is seriously ill and cannot eat on its own, feeding by a stomach tube may be necessary. If your veterinarian feels that you should use this method of force feeding, he or she will explain what equipment is necessary and demonstrate the correct way to pass the tube over the tongue and into the stomach.

Force-feed at intervals of 8 to 12 hours and stop forcing food as soon as the dog's appetite resumes.

Kitchen Hygiene

Kitchen hygiene is important to successful nursing. All bowls, force-feeding implements, or other utensils that come into contact with the patient should be washed in boiling soapy water, rinsed thoroughly, and dried. All rejected food should be thrown away. Food from partly used cans should be transferred to a clean dish, covered with plastic wrap, and refrigerated. Before this food is used, it should be brought to room temperature. Be sure to wash your hands after handling either the dog or feeding dishes or utensils that have come into contact with the dog.

HOW TO TAKE YOUR DOG'S TEMPERATURE

Since many infectious disorders begin with a fever, taking the temperature should be one of the first things you do when you suspect your dog is sick. Fever or elevated temperature may be accompanied by other symptoms, such as change in eating or drinking habits, change in urination or bowel movements, or just a general listlessness. Both temperature and other changes in your dog's condition should be reported to your veterinarian as soon as any illness is suspected. For convalescing dogs too, you can correctly determine if the animal has a fever only by taking its temperature. A warm nose or muzzle may indicate fever, but they are not accurate enough to rely on.

Taking a dog's temperature is not difficult. It should be measured rectally—not orally, since the dog can bite down and break the thermometer. Before inserting the rectal thermometer, hold the end (opposite the bulb) between your thumb and index finger, and using sharp, vigorous downward movements, shake the mercury column to below 95°F (35°C). Lubricate the bulb end with lubricating or petroleum jelly or baby oil. Place the dog on a firm surface, preferably standing with its hindquarters facing you (temperature can also be measured with the dog lying down). If the dog is uncooperative, tie a safety muzzle around its mouth before inserting the thermometer, to avoid being bitten. See "Handling and Restraint" in section I to learn how to tie a safety muzzle and the assistant's position if help is needed to control the dog.

Grasp the tail with your free hand to steady the dog. Push the thermometer gently into the rectum, bulb end first (Illus. 48). How far you insert the thermometer depends on the dog's size. An inch is enough for small breeds; 2 inches or so may be necessary for large breeds. Leave the thermometer in place 2 to 3 minutes. Hold the

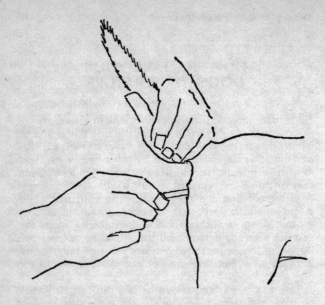

48. TAKING A DOG'S TEMPERATURE

opposite end of the thermometer steady and try to keep
the dog from sitting down. Remove the thermometer,
wipe it off with cotton or a tissue, and read the temperature.

How to Read the Thermometer

Once the thermometer has been removed and cleaned,
hold it between your thumb and index finger and roll it
back and forth until you locate the mercury column in
the center. The point at the end of the mercury is the
dog's temperature (Illus. 49).

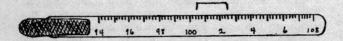

49. NORMAL TEMPERATURE OF DOG—100.5 TO 102.5

What Is a Normal Temperature?

A dog's normal rectal temperature is 100.5°F to 102.5°F (38°C to 39°C). An elevated temperature usually indicates disease, but not if the elevation is slight. Hot weather, excitement, exercise, and even digestion of food can cause a slight, temporary rise in temperature. When a dog appears to be sick, however, its temperature should be taken in the morning and in the evening, for this information will be valuable to your veterinarian. Elevation over 102.5°F (39°C) should be considered as fever. A temperature drop below 100°F (37°C), except in young puppies under 1 month of age, should be regarded as serious, calling for immediate treatment. Wrap the dog in blankets and get to a veterinarian as soon as possible.

Care of the Thermometer

After you have recorded the temperature, wash the thermometer in cold water, wipe it with rubbing alcohol, and place it inside its case. When you use the same thermometer on several pets, be sure to immerse it temporarily in rubbing alcohol after each use to prevent the passage of germs.

DETERMINING YOUR DOG'S HEARTBEAT AND PULSE

You can feel your dog's heartbeat on the lower part of the chest on the left side, just behind the elbow. Place your fingers or the palm of your hand on the chest near the elbow and move about until you can locate the beat through the chest wall. The heartbeat may be difficult to feel if your dog is obese or has a substantial chest wall, as in St. Bernards, Newfoundlands, and Bernese Mountain Dogs.

The best place to take your dog's pulse is over the femoral artery at the inside of the thigh on the back leg. Here, just below the point where the leg joins the body, the femoral artery crosses the thighbone and is near to the skin, making it easy for you to detect the pulse. The pulse rate can vary according to breed, age, and general

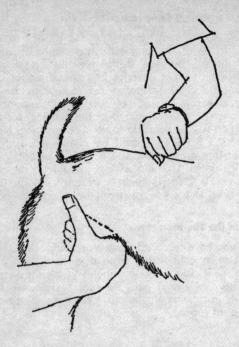

50. TAKING A DOG'S PULSE

health from 80 to 140 beats per minute. Generally, smaller dogs, especially toy breeds and puppies, have higher pulse rates than large dogs.

To take the pulse, place your index and middle fingers on the inside of the leg while your thumb presses on the outside (Illus. 50), and count the beats for 1 minute. If your dog refuses to remain still, count the beats for 15 seconds, then multiply by 4 to determine the rate per minute. Conditions that temporarily cause a slight rise in rectal temperature can also make the pulse rise temporarily.

It's a good idea to know your dog's normal pulse rate; then, when illness is suspected, it is easier to determine whether the pulse is higher or lower than normal, and whether the dog is in shock. The normal pulse is a steady and firm beat; a fast, shallow pulse is typical of shock.

DETERMINING
THE RESPIRATORY RATE

The respiratory rate of a healthy dog at rest is 10 to 30 breaths per minute. A relaxed dog breathes through its nose while the chest moves in a smooth, almost rhythmic manner. After excitement, heat, exercise, or certain types of stress, the respiratory rate increases. As the rate speeds up, the dogs tends to breathe through its mouth—and when respiration becomes very accelerated, the dog begins to pant. Dogs do not perspire like people who have sweat glands in nearly all parts of the body. In humans, sweating plays an important part in the regulation of body temperature. One of the ways a dog regulates body temperature is by panting.

To ascertain the respiratory rate, you should count either the exhalations (breathing out) or inhalations (breathing in) but not both. Try to learn the quality and rate of your dog's normal breathing at rest, and after excitement or exercise or during hot weather, so you will be able to determine when irregularities occur. This can be important when illness is suspected, especially in an emergency.

In life-threatening emergencies, you can always determine if the dog is breathing by holding a hair or thread in front of its nose. Even a limited degree of airflow can be observed by the movement of the thread.

HOW TO GIVE MEDICINES

Giving medicine to your dog can be one of the most unpleasant aspects of home nursing. However, there are times when medication is necessary for your pet's recovery and you must know the correct way to administer pills, capsules, liquids, and other medications without causing further trauma, especially if you are nursing the dog at home following surgery or a serious illness. Most dogs try to resist when they must swallow pills or liquids, but giving medicines does not have to be a harrowing experience when you know the correct procedures.

Giving Pills or Capsules

Small and medium-sized dogs should be seated on a sturdy surface (the top of a well-made table or your automatic clothes dryer will do nicely); large breeds should be seated against a wall so they cannot escape or back away.

The following directions are for a right-handed person; reverse them if you are left-handed. Lift the dog's head with your left hand and place the left palm on top of the dog's muzzle. The mouth will open if you grasp the upper jaw behind the canine teeth with your fingers on one side and thumb on the other and press the lips inward (Illus. 51). When the lips are held over the teeth this way, you should have no difficulty keeping the mouth open. The right hand is then free to administer the medication. Pick up the pill with your thumb and index finger (and use this hand to steady the lower jaw, if necessary). Place the tablet on the base of the tongue, well back in the throat, and push gently downward. Quickly withdraw your fingers and close the mouth. Keep the head upward at about a 45° angle until the pill or capsule is swallowed. If necessary, tickle the dog's throat to stimulate swallowing.

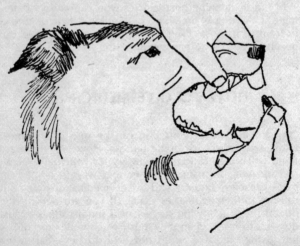

51. ADMINISTERING SOLID ORAL MEDICATION BY HAND

It's not too difficult to give a pill or capsule in this manner, but if the dog is fussy or if you don't place the pill far enough back on the tongue, the dog may be able to spit it out and you will have to repeat the procedure. If you experience difficulties, try coating the pill with butter or margarine, or covering it with cheese, liverwurst, ground meat, or some other food the dog finds appetizing. When giving large capsules to dogs, swallowing is easier if the medication is first coated with butter or margarine. If you are afraid to use your fingers to administer the pill, use a forceps to place the medication at the back of the tongue (Illus. 52).

If all else fails, crumble the tablet or empty the capsule contents into the dog's food and mix thoroughly, *but be sure your dog eats all its food*. This method is only a last resort, for it's almost impossible to deceive a dog even if the medication has been mixed thoroughly in the food. Enteric-coated tablets should not be taken apart before they are swallowed. They are specially coated with a substance that is dissolved only by intestinal enzymes.

If assistance is needed to control the dog, see "Handling and Restraint" in section I.

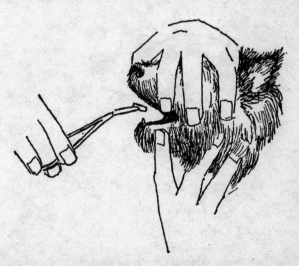

52. ADMINISTERING SOLID ORAL MEDICATION BY FORCEPS

Giving Liquids by the Lip-Pocket Method

Liquids are best given to a dog by:
1. A medicine bottle with a narrow cap
2. A medicine dropper (made of plastic, not glass)
3. A spillproof spoon made for giving liquid medicines to infants. These are usually calibrated from $1/4$ teaspoonful to 2 tablespoonsful.

Remember: Before giving liquid suspensions, always shake well to evenly distribute the contents.

Never open a dog's mouth and try to pour liquid medicine down the throat. The correct way to administer liquids is the lip-pocket method. Place your thumb and index finger at the corner of the mouth, where the dog's upper and lower lip join. Gently pull the skin outward and downward to form a pocket between the teeth and lips (Illus. 53). Raise the dog's head slightly and slowly pour the liquid medicine into the pocket where it should pass easily between the teeth and down the throat. If the dog keeps the liquid in its mouth, massage the throat to induce swallowing. While the head should be held upward until all the liquid is swallowed, it should not be held so high as to interfere with the natural swallowing process.

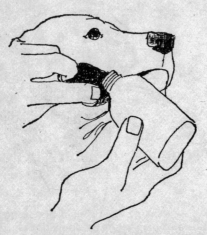

53. ADMINISTERING LIQUID ORAL MEDICATION
BY LIP-POCKET METHOD

A plastic kitchen poultry baster or syringe is another convenient way to administer liquid medicine to dogs, especially medium and large breeds. Once the baster or syringe is filled, place its opening in the pocket between the lips and teeth (Illus. 54), then slowly squeeze the baster or depress the syringe plunger to allow the liquid to enter the mouth.

If the dog has a bad disposition, an assistant may be necessary to help restrain it. (See "Handling and Restraint" in section I.) A safety muzzle can be used, providing it is tied loosely enough to permit the jaws to open and allow swallowing once the liquid has been poured into the pocket of the dog's mouth.

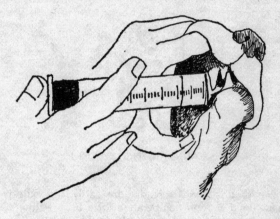

54. ADMINISTERING LIQUID ORAL MEDICATION BY SYRINGE

APPLYING TOPICAL MEDICATIONS

Medicating the Eyes

If the eyes have a discharge, they should be cleaned before any ophthalmic medication is applied. Dampen a piece of sterile cotton or a cotton ball with warm water and wipe away any mucus which has accumulated in the inner corners of the eyes. *Do not rub over the eyeball, for you can scratch the eye or cause an irritation.*

Eye drops should be applied like this:

1. Tilt the dog's head upward and backward with your hand (Illus. 55), while using the thumb of this hand to open the lower lid.
2. Hold the dropper or bottle in your other hand, steadying this hand on the dog's head to prevent eye injury if the pet should move suddenly.
3. Drop the prescribed amount of medication into the inner corner of the eye(s).
4. Wipe away any excess solution under the eyes with cotton.

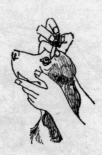

55. ADMINISTERING EYE DROPS

Eye ointment will spread more easily and quickly if maintained at room temperature (or a little warmer) before application. Apply eye ointment like this:

1. Raise the dog's head upward and backward.
2. Use your thumb to pull the lower lid slightly outward and downward to separate it from the eyeball (Illus. 56).
3. Holding the tube in your other hand, squeeze a fine ribbon of ointment into the space between the lower lid and lower part of the eye.
4. Allow the lid to go back into place. As the dog opens and closes its eyelids, the ointment will melt and coat the entire eye.

Be careful that the end of the dropper bottle or ointment tube does not touch the eye, for this can contaminate the ophthalmic medication.

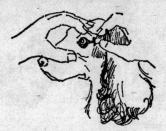

56. ADMINISTERING EYE OINTMENT

Medicating the Ears

If your dog's ears become infected, the veterinarian may prescribe ointment or liquid medication to be placed in the ear canal. Before inserting any medication, use a piece of sterile cotton or cotton ball to clean out any wax, dirt, or old medication which may have accumulated in the canal. (See "Grooming: Cleaning the Ears" in section IV for the correct way to clean the ears.) Most ear medication is easy to apply: ointments usually are packaged in tubes with long, thin nozzles for convenient application into the ear canal; liquids usually come packed in dropper bottles. Use this method to apply ear medication:

1. If the dog is a breed with hanging ears, draw the earflaps backward, close to the head.

2. Take hold of the cartilage at the base of the ear (Illus. 57), and draw it straight out from the dog's head. In this position, any liquid or ointment inserted in the ear will flow directly into the canal, ensuring proper medication.

3. Drop the required amount of liquid or squeeze the necessary amount of ointment into the ear canal.

4. Lower the earflap (if necessary) and temporarily steady the head with your hand to keep the dog from shaking.

5. Use your other hand to gently massage the base of the ear to help distribute the medication inside.

6. Release your hold on the dog's muzzle. Use cotton to absorb any excess liquid.

215

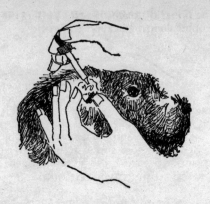

57. MEDICATING EAR

As soon as you release your hold on the muzzle, the dog will probably shake its head. Don't be concerned. This is just nature's way of protecting the delicate structure of the ear canal.

GIVING INJECTIONS

While it is uncommon for a pet owner to have to give injections, there are certain conditions, diabetes for example, where drugs have to be taken into the dog's body, not through its digestive tract but subcutaneously (under the skin), intramuscularly, or intravenously (into a vein), by means of a syringe and needle. Usually this is done by a veterinarian; if it is ever necessary to give your dog an injection at home, the procedure must be done under the supervision and instruction of your veterinarian.

Injections should be given in as sterile a manner as possible by someone who is well trained. A veterinarian should demonstrate the step-by-step procedures involved, so that you become familiar with correct techniques. An injection that is given carelessly or incorrectly can seriously harm the patient. *Remember that it is unlawful to have needles and syringes in your possession unless they have been prescribed by a physician or veterinarian.*

GUIDELINES FOR THE USE
OF MEDICATIONS

Many illnesses require treatment by medications. The pet owner who cares for a sick or convalescent dog and assumes the responsibility of giving medications can follow the veterinarian's instructions better when he or she knows how to give the drug safely, what precautions should be observed, and what results can be expected. Treatment will be more successful if the pet owner and veterinarian keep each other fully informed during the healing process.

Drugs must be prescribed by a veterinarian, who is the only qualified person to determine appropriate medication. But once the medication has been prescribed, the pet owner and veterinarian must exchange information that will be vital to the dog's recovery. Here are guidelines for the pet owner:

1. Learn the name of the prescribed drug and how it will change the diagnosed condition.

2. Know the correct dosage schedule, that is, how often the medicine should be given, and follow it as closely as possible. Don't miss a dose and double the prescribed portion the next time. Some dogs are fussy when they have to take medicine and it's easy for an owner to become discouraged and give the remedy "hit or miss." A battle does not have to take place between dog and owner! As previously mentioned, many tricks can be used to give medicines; with a little experimentation, one of them should be successful.

3. Learn when the medication should be given. Should the dog take it before meals, after meals, or if the dog is extremely fussy, can it be mixed with food as a last resort? Certain drugs (those of the Penicillin and Tetracyline families) are better absorbed if taken 1 hour before or 2 hours after eating.

4. Know if any special precautions should be observed. Can foods, liquids, exercise, other medicines, or mild exposure to the sun or cold alter the effects of the drug? For example, dairy products are known to interfere with the absorption of Tetracycline, so that milk should be avoided for 1 hour before and after each dose.

5. Learn about possible side effects or adverse reactions. Among undesirable results a side effect is an expected response that accompanies the desirable action of the drug, and an adverse reaction is an unexpected effect —which may be dangerous, even life-threatening. Check with your veterinarian and learn which drug-caused symptoms should be reported immediately. The degree of the side effects can often be lessened by reducing the dosage or by substituting another drug of the same family.

6. Find out how long the medication should be given to the dog.

7. Learn how much time should elapse before reporting to the veterinarian significant or no change in the dog's condition.

8. Do not stop the medication just because you feel your dog is getting better.

9. Determine if another appointment is necessary. Does the dog need a follow-up examination to determine the effects of the medication?

10. Should the prescription be refilled? If so, how often, and why?

11. If there is anything confusing about your dog's medication, ask your veterinarian to clarify his instructions. *Your dog's life may depend on them.*

In conclusion, do remember to:

1. Give medication selected or prescribed by your veterinarian
2. Follow prescribed dosage schedules as closely as possible
3. Inform your veterinarian immediately if you think the medication is causing an adverse reaction
4. Store the medication out of the reach of the dog and children, to avoid accidental poisoning
5. Throw away outdated drugs. Don't use medication that was prescribed for a previous illness
6. Keep a written record of all drugs and vaccines administered:
   name, dosage, dates, and reasons for use
7. Keep a written record of any medication to which your dog becomes allergic or experiences serious side effects. Inform your veterinarian beforehand of all aller-

218

gies or adverse reactions and be sure this information is placed on your dog's medical record

HOW TO GIVE AN ENEMA

Constipation is an occasional problem of small animals. (See "Constipation" in section I.) It may be necessary to give an enema to relieve the condition by emptying the bowels of impacted matter. If the dog is recovering from a serious illness or operation, consult with your veterinarian before giving an enema. He may wish to prescribe a mild laxative or infant suppository first.

Preparing the Patient

If your dog is not recovering from an illness or operation and has enough strength to resist, an assistant may be necessary to help restrain the dog while the enema is being given. Most convalescent dogs will be too feeble to put up a fight, but remember to tie a gauze safety muzzle around the mouth if the dog tries to bite. (See "Handling and Restraint" in section I.) If the dog is profusely coated, trimming off some of the hair around the anus beforehand will make the results less messy.

Carefully select where to give the enema. It can be outdoors on a grassy lawn in warm weather (for a healthy dog, of course) or indoors in the basement, in a bathtub—or for small breeds and puppies, on top of a firm surface. Whatever place you choose, prepare the area in advance by putting down a supply of newspapers.

Steps in Giving an Enema

Ideally the enema should be administered with the dog standing, but it can lie on its side if necessary. A disposable enema for humans, such as the Fleet®, is effective for dogs and convenient to administer. A disposable enema is packaged in an easy-grip squeeze bottle with prelubricated top and can be purchased at most pharmacies in either adult or pediatric size.

An enema should be given as gently as possible. Bring the disposable enema to room temperature or warmer. Remove the protective shield, and with steady pressure, gently insert the tip into the rectum. Squeeze the contents slowly, using about 1 to $1\frac{1}{2}$ ounces per 10 pounds of body weight. When the correct amount of liquid has been expelled from the bottle, withdraw the top from the rectum. Steady the dog on the papers. Results should be obtained immediately.

You can prepare your own enema solution instead of using a disposable product. Prompt relief of constipation is usually obtained when warm soapy water enemas are given. Add about 1 ounce of Ivory or other mild soap that does not contain detergent per quart of warm water. The soapy water mixture should be inserted into the rectum by means of an enema bag or gravity flow apparatus. Fill the enema bag with the soapy water mixture; shut the hose clamp and elevate the bag. Lubricate the nozzle with Vaseline® or other lubricating jelly. Insert the tip into the rectum, unclamp the hose, and slowly begin to administer the liquid. If you encounter a fecal mass, gently move the nozzle back and forth until the liquid breaks the mass apart. Administer about 3 to 4 ounces of liquid for small breeds and puppies, as much as 1 pint for medium-sized breeds like Cocker Spaniels and Miniature Poodles, and about 1 quart for large breeds. As you give the enema, speak quietly and reassuringly to your dog, as it may be frightened.

Either kind of enema can be repeated; but if the impaction is not relieved after two enemas, consult your veterinarian.

After the dog has its bowel movement, roll up the soiled newspapers and clean the area. If its hindquarters have a foul odor or are soiled with feces, wash the hair with shampoo and water, then rinse thoroughly. The coat should be dried completely, especially if the dog is recovering from an illness. The cleaning should take place immediately after the bowel movement, for if pieces of stool are allowed to harden in the coat, they will be difficult to remove later on.

If the thought of giving an enema seems unpleasant, try using glycerin suppositories. Infant suppositories are easy to use on dogs because of their long, thin shape.

Insert the suppository in the rectum and hold it in place, if necessary, following the manufacturer's directions.

BANDAGES

Various dressings and bandages are described in "Your Dog's First-Aid Kit" in section I. Application of dressings and bandages for emergencies and minor wounds are described fully at "Bandaging" in section I.

If a sick dog requires complicated dressings and bandages, it will usually stay in the hospital as long as they are necessary. If your dog is recuperating at home after surgery or a serious injury and complicated bandages are necessary, several precautions should be observed. The complicated dressing and bandage may become loose or be bitten or pulled off by the dog.

1. Should the wound begin bleeding profusely, this should be considered an emergency situation. Control the bleeding with pressure bandages as instructed at "Bleeding" in section I.

2. If there is no bleeding, temporarily rebandage the area to prevent contamination.

3. Consult your veterinarian as soon as possible. Never attempt to redress a complicated dressing and bandage without professional advice.

As healing progresses, the dog may try to scratch, bite, or rub the bandaged part in an attempt to get at the wound. Tips to prevent self-mutilation are included at the end of "Bandaging" in section I.

COLLECTING FECAL AND URINE SAMPLES

To diagnose certain diseases, your veterinarian may examine a sample of the dog's feces or urine.

How to Collect Fecal Samples

Collecting a fecal sample for the veterinarian is not difficult. Once the dog has moved its bowels, pick up a sample and transfer it to a clean, closed container or seal it in plastic wrap or a plastic sandwich bag. If the movement occurs outdoors, try not to accumulate grass, dirt, or other objects in the sample you collect. Print your name and address on a label and attach it to the sample for proper identification.

The stool sample should be fresh. Especially when being microscopically inspected for the presence of internal parasite eggs, the sample should be examined within 3 hours after it is collected. Refrigerate the sample if it will be stored at home for several hours. Heat or procrastination in delivering the sample to your veterinarian may cause parasite eggs to mature and burst, making identification difficult.

How to Collect Urine Samples

Collecting a urine sample demands a bit more determination from the pet owner. To gather a urine specimen, us a clean, dry container: a wide-mouthed jar, pie pan, or small disposable baking pan. Attach the dog's collar and lead for control and go outside (if the dog's health permits). As soon as a female squats or a male lifts his leg, place the container underneath to collect some urine. Don't worry about capturing the entire stream of urine: 2 to 3 ounces is enough for analysis.

An early morning urine sample is preferred, because it will be concentrated and contain ingredients important for analysis. When the sample has been collected, transfer it to a clean, dry bottle. Label the bottle with your name and address, then take it for analysis as soon as possible. Refrigerate the sample if it will be kept at home for a few hours.

Remember that the healing process may be prolonged; when the dog first comes home from the hospital, it may need round-the-clock care. Be sure you can carry out the doctor's orders and give your dog every chance to recover. Competent nursing and plenty of tender loving care play an important part in how quickly your dog will get well.

Section III

BREEDING
AND
REPRODUCTION

BREEDING PROS AND CONS

The decision to breed your bitch requires a great deal of thought. Raising a litter of puppies sounds like fun, but the whelping and care of a litter is not only time-consuming, but can be expensive. Then you may not be able to find suitable homes for the puppies. Before you make the decision to breed your bitch, consider the following questions:

Why Do You Want to Breed?

It is often said that breeding is beneficial for a female, that it improves health and temperament, and that every bitch should have the experience of raising a litter of puppies. There is little evidence to support these theories. Many bitches make wonderful mothers, but others find whelping a frightening episode. After whelping a litter, some dams refuse to accept or nurse their puppies. If you are breeding only to have your bitch experience motherhood, you are imposing human mores on your dog. Then again, how many times have you heard people say that they are breeding their bitches just to allow their children to watch "the miracle of birth"? Of course, if you own a fine purebred bitch from a line of great dogs and want to continue a breeding program to produce quality puppies, by all means do so, but don't breed just because you believe it will be good for your dog or educational for your children!

Can You Afford to Breed?

Never breed a dog with the expectation of making money. The thought of selling puppies at high prices may be attractive, but the hidden expenses in breeding and whelping a litter can be high. You may have to pay for stud service (in cash); veterinarian's expenses (including pre-breeding examination, examination before whelping, treatment for possible whelping complications, and post-whelping attention to the dam and puppies); additional food for the dam and her puppies; registering the litter with the American Kennel Club (AKC); advertising the puppies for sale; inoculations for the puppies; etc. Expect to spend money for at least 4 months before you get any money from puppy sales.

Do You Have Adequate Space to Raise a Litter?

This requires a great deal of consideration, especially if your bitch is of a large breed. It is necessary to decide where the litter will be born and allow the bitch to become secure in her quarters.

Once the litter has been born, the mother and her puppies will stay in one location for about 3 weeks. After the third week, as the puppies begin to become more active and interested in their surroundings, the family can be relocated to another area, such as a quiet, warm corner of the kitchen or den, where the puppies can be with their mother but also learn to socialize, that is, can have free play with their littermates as well as playing with and being handled by humans. As long as there is space to exercise and play, small-breed puppies present no problems at 6 weeks of age; however, medium and large-sized puppies become very active by age 4 to 6 weeks and it is difficult to keep them confined in a small area for long.

Do You Have the Time and Energy to Raise Puppies?

The breeding and whelping of your bitch and rearing of the puppies will take about 4 months of your time—possibly longer, if the puppies are difficult to sell. You must make a commitment to be available, beginning with the bitch's last weeks of pregnancy. You must be present at whelping time, when it may be necessary to help the bitch, or if complications occur, to get her quickly to a veterinarian. Once the puppies are born, it may not be difficult for you for the first 3 weeks if the mother feeds and cares for them. But should she be unable to or refuse to, because of a postwhelping complication, you may have to hand-raise the litter. Will you be prepared and have the patience to hand-feed the entire litter every 3 to 4 hours?

Raising a litter is hard work, especially after weaning time. Puppies are darling and cuddly, but they also can be sloppy and dirty—they overturn feeding dishes and sit in their food; they vomit; they tramp around in bowel movements—and *you* must clean them!

Interviewing prospective buyers by phone and in person involves a lot of time. Each time a prospective buyer comes, the dam and her puppies have to be in fresh condition for viewing. Can you handle this? Consider your emotional involvement with the puppies, too. You can't sell them to just anybody! You must be sure each puppy will receive love and the best of care from its new owner.

Can You Find Suitable Homes for the Puppies?

Many puppies and kittens are put to sleep at an early age in humane shelters every year because there are no homes for them. Dogs and cats are suffering from overpopulation throughout the world. Each hour in the United States 415 human babies are born; during the same hour, 10,000 to 15,000 puppies and kittens are born.* Only a small percentage of these helpless animals will find homes, so in order to keep a stable pet population, thousands of dogs and cats must die each day.

Animal control figures are shocking. The Humane Society of the United States estimates that 12 million to 15 million dogs and cats are put to sleep each year. There is a misconception that animals put to sleep in pounds are only mongrels, but while many mixed-breeds are handled in animal shelters, so are many purebreds— Irish Setters and German Shepherds are among the most common. These are not just lost dogs that have been picked up by humane officers, but dogs that have been turned in by people who know they will be euthanized, not adopted. Finally, the figures cited represent only the animals handled by the various humane groups. Humane workers estimate that twice as many animals never make it to shelters—instead, they are killed on streets or in fields, they starve or freeze or are destroyed by their owners—as are euthanized.

To breed a mixed-breed dog is especially inhumane. A popular rationalization is that "it would be nice to keep

* Based on estimates by the Humane Society of the United States.

one of Spot's puppies." It's not fair to the puppy to expect it to be an exact replica of a mixed-breed mother. So if Spot is a mixed-breed, have her spayed, let her live a happy life, and after she passes away, if you think you are able to care for another dog, get one. The world and especially the humane shelters are overflowing with dogs —each one asking for love and attention and the right to live.

The preceding is not meant to frighten the prospective breeder, though it probably has. But if we have made you realize that there is a serious pet overpopulation problem and that while breeding a bitch and rearing a litter may seem a delightful thing to do, it requires a great deal of patience, responsibility, and time on your part, we have accomplished a great deal.

THE CONDITION OF THE MOTHER-TO-BE

If you decide to breed your bitch, pay attention to her general condition. The prospective dam should be in good physical shape (not too fat or too thin), to increase not only the possibility of conception but of delivering healthy puppies and caring for them until weaning.

Is the bitch too thin? This may be caused by inadequate nutrition or internal or external parasites. Is she too fat? This can be caused by incorrect diet, metabolic problems, or lack of exercise. Consult your veterinarian about correcting her weight, to avoid complications.

What is the condition of the bitch's skin and hair? Is the skin soft and supple and the hair lustrous (indications of good overall health), or is she infested with fleas or ticks? Take immediate steps to rid the bitch of external parasites and learn how to prevent reinfestation.

Was your bitch ever injured in an automobile or other serious accident? If so, have her reexamined thoroughly by a veterinarian before mating, especially if the injuries were in the pelvic area.

Anyone who is planning to breed should take the prospective mother to a veterinarian for a complete examination 1 to 2 months before she is due to be in heat.

Problems such as internal and external parasites, skin problems, infected teeth, infections, vaginal discharge, and weight problems should be treated and corrected by mating time. Make sure that her boosters for distemper, hepatitis, and leptospirosis are up to date.

WHEN TO BREED

Male dogs often become sexually interested at 5 to 6 months old, but they are not able to reproduce until they are about 10 months old. The female's ability to reproduce is determined by a heat cycle which lasts about 21 days and may start soon after the age of 6 months; many bitches, however, are age 12 months or more before they have their first heat cycle. Once a bitch has been in season, she usually comes into season every 5 to 7 months. (Some females come into heat only once in every 9 to 12 months.)

If your bitch is between 6 and 12 months old when she has her first season, it is wise to wait for the second (or later) season. If your bitch has her first season at 14 to 18 months of age or later, she may be bred, providing that she is physically and mentally mature. It depends on the particular bitch and her breed. Seek your veterinarian's advice about the correct age to breed, particularly with large and giant breeds where it may be wise to wait until the third season (about 2 years of age) when the bitch will be fully grown and mature in other respects.

THE HEAT CYCLE

Novice breeders are often confused about when to breed a bitch. Without getting too technical, this is what happens during the female's heat period which lasts about 21 days:

The first signs are swelling of the vulva, and usually several days later, a blood-tinged discharge. This first stage is called proestrus (or preheat) and lasts about 9 days after the blood discharge begins. Males are attracted to the bitch, but usually she is not yet interested in breeding.

The second stage, called estrus, starts around the 9th day of the heat and continues for the next 7 to 10 days, during which time ovulation occurs. Now the bitch usually will allow a male to breed her. Many bitches continue bleeding during estrus; in others, the discharge may slow down or stop during this stage. The most suitable time for mating is from the 9th to the 12th day, when the vulva becomes less swollen and spongy to the touch and the discharge changes to a light pink or straw color. There are exceptions; not all bitches breed on the same days. Some are ready for mating earlier than the 9th day while others may not be ready until after the 12th day.

Keep a close check on the bitch to help determine when she is ready. Besides observing vulva sponginess and discharge color, you can lightly touch the vulva with your index finger. If the bitch whips her tail to one side, she probably is ready to be bred. The best indication is the bitch's behavior with the stud dog. She will not stand for breeding if she is not ready, and most experienced stud dogs are not seriously interested in a bitch that will not stand.

THE STUD DOG

Choose the stud dog before your bitch is due to come in season. See "For Additional Reading: Breeding and Reproduction" at the end of the book for more information about choosing a stud dog.

The stud dog owner receives a fee, which may be a cash payment at time of mating (the amount depends on the dog's pedigree, show record, quality of previous litters sired, etc.) or may be an agreement that the stud's owner can choose a puppy when the litter are 6 to 8 weeks old. Arrangements should be incorporated in a written stud service contract and signed by both parties. The contract does not need to be complicated, but it should contain basic information that will protect both sides: for example, the names of the two dogs, AKC registration numbers, date(s) of mating(s), and stud-fee terms.

If a puppy is promised, specify if it will be the pick of the litter and at what age it is to be selected. If the stud fee is paid in cash, the contract should guarantee a repeat breeding (without charge) if there are no puppies.

At the time of breeding the bitch is taken to the male, primarily because the male does most of the work and is more likely to feel confident and dominant in familiar surroundings.

When you present your bitch for breeding, don't be offended if the stud's owners want to steady her (or ask you to steady her) during the mating or to muzzle her if she snaps. *Matings must always be observed or supervised. Breeding is not done by putting both dogs in a room and shutting the door!* It is customary for the bitch to be bred twice within a 48-hour period.

BREEDING

When you present your bitch for breeding, she and the stud dog should be allowed to get acquainted and to conduct a few minutes of "flirtation" before they are mated. When the actual breeding takes place, the bitch may cry out—usually from stimulation and not from pain. It is possible, however, for a maiden bitch to experience fleeting discomfort when the dog's penis first penetrates and swells, but usually this passes quickly.

After penetration, the male will make several thrusting motions and then become tied to the bitch. This involves the bulb at the base of the male's penis and a sphincter muscle ring in the female's vagina. After insertion, the sheath of the penis is pulled back behind the bulb and the penis becomes congested with blood. As the bulb passes the ring, the sphincter muscles hold it so firmly that the animals become temporarily tied together and cannot separate. Now the male's semen is being ejaculated.

A tie can last 5 to 60 minutes, averaging 15 to 20 minutes. Usually after the tie begins the dog will turn one hind leg over the bitch's back and the pair will stand rear to rear (like the dogs in Illus. 58) until the tie releases. The swelling of the genitalia reduces gradually,

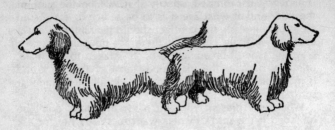

58. BREEDING; THE TIE

but when separation comes it comes quickly. After breeding, keep your bitch quiet and keep other males away from her until her heat cycle is completed.

MISMATING

The female, ready for breeding around the middle of the heat period, can be quite eager to accept a male. If a male can't get to her, she may try to get to him. Therefore, if you do not wish to have your bitch bred, she should be confined indoors during her season. Her movements outside should be supervised (always on lead) and she should not be allowed to run free until the heat cycle is finished. Some commercially available products, such as Ring 5 Femme Tabs, can help to counteract the female mating odors that attract male dogs. They are palatable tablets that can be fed orally or crushed and mixed with food; they do not alter the normal heat cycle, are not birth-control pills, and do not reduce the desire for breeding. Birth-control pills for dogs are available through veterinarians; consult yours for additional information.

Misalliances can happen: occasionally a bitch will get out and be bred. Male dogs can be very persistent too; when a bitch is in heat, they will make every effort to reach her, digging under or climbing fences, breeding through fences, or squeezing through the tiniest openings. The male cannot withdraw his penis until the tie between the couple subsides naturally. To forcibly separate the pair can cause serious physical damage to them. In the event of a mismating:

1. Do not attempt to break the tie.
2. Do not hose or pour water over the dogs. Do not hit or otherwise abuse either of the dogs: it is inhumane and will not help separate the pair any faster.
3. Allow the tie between the pair to release naturally.
4. Vaginal douching after mating is practically useless, since the sperm entered the uterus before the breeding was completed.
5. Take the bitch to your veterinarian as soon as possible for hormone treatment to prevent pregnancy. The veterinarian will give her an injection and possibly prescribe medication to be given at home. The purpose of this treatment is to extend the bleeding and keep the fertilized egg from becoming attached to the lining of the uterus. Don't procrastinate! Treatment is effective when given within 24 hours after the mating. *Caution:* This treatment will prolong the heat cycle a week or 2 longer than usual and you must continue to confine your bitch until the cycle is finished so another mismating will not occur.
6. The hormone treatment may not be effective, in which case your alternatives are:
   a. To have your veterinarian perform an ovariohysterectomy (spaying) as soon as the heat cycle is completed;
   b. To have a cesarean section performed late in the pregnancy and have the puppies removed. This is a traumatic experience for the bitch, however, and not recommended by most veterinarians.
   c. To wait and see if the bitch is pregnant, and if she is, to allow her to have the puppies.

FALSE PREGNANCY

False pregnancy (pseudopregnancy) is confusing to most dog owners. It appears in a female 6 to 8 weeks after the heat cycle, even though no breeding has occurred. The signs of false pregancy are barely noticeable in some bitches, but very apparent in others.

233

Physical signs can range from a slight swelling of the breasts with a slight watery secretion, to noticeable abdominal swelling and enlarged breasts which produce milk. Emotionally, the bitch begins to act as though she were pregnant, scratching rugs, newspapers, or blankets, or rearranging her own bedding to prepare a "nest" for her puppies. She may lose her appetite, have a tendency to sleep much more, and try to hide in secluded places, in a closet or under the bed. As "whelping" time approaches, she may cry, be quite restless, and even simulate the process of giving birth. Often the bitch will believe that one of her toys, a slipper, or some other soft object is her puppy. She will carry it around and act very possessively toward the object, putting it in the nest and expecting it to nurse on her breasts.

If the symptoms of false pregnancy are not severe, the female usually recovers from this state naturally within a week or so. If the signs are severe, consult your veterinarian as soon as possible. If there is a great deal of milk production, try not to rub or "milk" the breasts for relief, as this will only cause an increase in the flow. A temporary reduction of food and liquid intake often helps decrease milk production. *If the breasts become hot, swollen, hard, or discolored, call your veterinarian immediately.* When a bitch has had one pseudopregnancy she may experience others after each subsequent heat cycle. In chronic cases, your veterinarian may suggest hormone treatment or that the bitch be bred. After the puppies are born, however, this does not guarantee that she will not have false pregnancies again. If a chronic female is not a valuable breeding bitch and you do not wish to raise a litter of puppies, you should consider having her spayed.

PRENATAL CARE

The average length of pregnancy (the gestation period), from mating to whelping, is 63 days. This can vary several days on account of breed (small dogs often whelp earlier than large breeds), number of puppies in the

234

litter, environmental conditions, and whether the bitch has whelped a previous litter.

For the first few weeks of pregnancy, if the bitch is being fed a balanced diet and receives sufficient, not too strenuous exercise, no change is necessary in her normal routine.

Signs of pregnancy depend on the size and physical condition of your bitch. They include:

1. Enlarged abdomen: This will be apparent about the 5th week and usually is observed as the flanks begin filling out. If the bitch is carrying only one or two puppies, enlargement of the abdomen may not be noticeable until late in her pregnancy.

2. Weight gain: There is not much of a weight gain during the first 4 weeks, but gain of 2 pounds in small bitches to 10 to 12 pounds in large bitches is possible during the last half of pregnancy. *An enlarged abdomen and weight gain can be caused by conditions such as pyrometra (infection of the uterus) or growths in the abdominal cavity, which may be confused with pregnancy.*

3. Changes in nipples and breasts: About the 35th day, the nipples begin to swell and stand out; they may appear to be very pink. As pregnancy advances, the breasts soften and gradually enlarge until about the 50th day, when the increase in size becomes very apparent. Several days before whelping, a watery liquid may be expressed from the nipples. Some of these signs can appear in a nonpregnant bitch during a false pregnancy.

4. Changes in temperament: Bitches usually become more serene, settled, and affectionate as pregnancy advances, but the occasional high-strung bitch may become more excitable or tense.

5. Movement of the abdomen: In the last 7 to 9 days of pregnancy, the unborn puppies can often be seen or touched as they move inside the bitch while she is lying in a relaxed position.

Any or all of these signs can be observed during the last part of pregnancy. If you need an earlier pregnancy diagnosis, at the 28th to 30th day of the gestation period, the presence of fetuses in the uterine horn can be demonstrated by palpating the abdomen, unless the bitch is large or overweight. Abdominal palpation should be done by a veterinarian, not by an untrained person—damage to the fetuses could result. Pregnancy can also be determined by an abdominal X ray after the 49th day.

REABSORPTION

Occasionally a bitch will show positive signs of pregnancy and then suddenly appear not to be pregnant. If the pregnancy is interrupted before the 4th or 5th week of gestation, it is possible for the bitch's body to reabsorb the developing fetuses. To determine that reabsorption has occurred, you must be certain that the bitch was pregnant and did not abort the puppies.

ABORTION—CANINE BRUCELLOSIS

Bitches abort their puppies occasionally. A bacterial disease of dogs, canine brucellosis, causes abortion near the end of pregnancy. The organism *Brucella canis* is spread by contact with the male during mating; with aborted fetuses; with an infectious vaginal discharge; with the feces of an infected animal; with breast secretions after an abortion; or with an infected substance that is eaten. Beagles are most often involved; canine brucellosis has also been diagnosed in Weimaraners, Greyhounds, Labrador Retrievers, Old English Sheepdogs, and Pointers and other breeds.

Once inside the body, the bacteria multiply rapidly and can be transported through the bloodstream of pregnant bitches to the placental tissues where they will infect the unborn fetuses.

Brucella canis causes abortions after the 30th day, and especially in the 7th to 9th weeks of pregnancy. If the embryos die early, they may be reabsorbed. When this happens, at whelping time there may be a dark, foul-smelling vaginal discharge. Or litters may be delivered with some puppies alive and others dead.

Specific antibodies can be found in the animal's bloodstream after infection: your veterinarian can determine the presence of *Brucella canis* by means of a serum agglutination test and blood cultures.

A mucid, greenish vaginal discharge is a common sign of abortion, which can occur from other causes. Consult your veterinarian as soon as possible.

FINAL WEEKS OF PREGNANCY

During the 4th week you should begin to gradually increase the bitch's food intake. Nutritionists agree that pregnancy and lactation are the most critical stress periods in a female dog's life: she requires increased levels of vitamins, minerals, amino acids, and energy, and if these are not received from an adequate diet, the bitch will get them by depleting her body reserves.

As the bitch's appetite and food intake increase, start offering two meals a day instead of one. As the pregnancy advances and the uterus enlarges, you may want to further divide her daily food intake into three or four meals to avoid feeding too much at one time. Nutritious additions to the diet include foods that contain a high level of protein, such as cottage cheese, cooked eggs, meat, and liver. Remember to provide fresh water at all times. Addition of a vitamin and mineral supplement, calcium, cod liver oil, and the like should be reserved for the advice of your veterinarian.

In the last half of pregnancy, exercise is important—not too strenuous, but adequate to maintain good muscle tone. Walks on leash are excellent but overactivity, especially running, jumping, and vigorous play periods with other pets or children, should be avoided. Toward the end of the pregnancy, be careful that the bitch does not become constipated.

While your bitch will appreciate a little extra love and attention during pregnancy, do not overindulge her. Bitches that have been spoiled during the gestation period may become so helpless and dependent on their owners that they refuse to accept their puppies after whelping.

Bred January	Due to whelp March	Bred February	Due to whelp April	Bred March	Due to whelp May	Bred April	Due to whelp June	Bred May	Due to whelp July	Bred June	Due to whelp August	Bred July	Due to whelp September	Bred August	Due to whelp October	Bred September	Due to whelp November	Bred October	Due to whelp December	Bred November	Due to whelp January	Bred December	Due to whelp February
1	5	1	5	1	3	1	3	1	3	1	3	1	2	1	3	1	3	1	3	1	3	1	2
2	6	2	6	2	4	2	4	2	4	2	4	2	3	2	4	2	4	2	4	2	4	2	3
3	7	3	7	3	5	3	5	3	5	3	5	3	4	3	5	3	5	3	5	3	5	3	4
4	8	4	8	4	6	4	6	4	6	4	6	4	5	4	6	4	6	4	6	4	6	4	5
5	9	5	9	5	7	5	7	5	7	5	7	5	6	5	7	5	7	5	7	5	7	5	6
6	10	6	10	6	8	6	8	6	8	6	8	6	7	6	8	6	8	6	8	6	8	6	7
7	11	7	11	7	9	7	9	7	9	7	9	7	8	7	9	7	9	7	9	7	9	7	8
8	12	8	12	8	10	8	10	8	10	8	10	8	9	8	10	8	10	8	10	8	10	8	9
9	13	9	13	9	11	9	11	9	11	9	11	9	10	9	11	9	11	9	11	9	11	9	10
10	14	10	14	10	12	10	12	10	12	10	12	10	11	10	12	10	12	10	12	10	12	10	11
11	15	11	15	11	13	11	13	11	13	11	13	11	12	11	13	11	13	11	13	11	13	11	12
12	16	12	16	12	14	12	14	12	14	12	14	12	13	12	14	12	14	12	14	12	14	12	13
13	17	13	17	13	15	13	15	13	15	13	15	13	14	13	15	13	15	13	15	13	15	13	14
14	18	14	18	14	16	14	16	14	16	14	16	14	15	14	16	14	16	14	16	14	16	14	15
15	19	15	19	15	17	15	17	15	17	15	17	15	16	15	17	15	17	15	17	15	17	15	16
16	20	16	20	16	18	16	18	16	18	16	18	16	17	16	18	16	18	16	18	16	18	16	17
17	21	17	21	17	19	17	19	17	19	17	19	17	18	17	19	17	19	17	19	17	19	17	18
18	22	18	22	18	20	18	20	18	20	18	20	18	19	18	20	18	20	18	20	18	20	18	19
19	23	19	23	19	21	19	21	19	21	19	21	19	20	19	21	19	21	19	21	19	21	19	20
20	24	20	24	20	22	20	22	20	22	20	22	20	21	20	22	20	22	20	22	20	22	20	21
21	25	21	25	21	23	21	23	21	23	21	23	21	22	21	23	21	23	21	23	21	23	21	22
22	26	22	26	22	24	22	24	22	24	22	24	22	23	22	24	22	24	22	24	22	24	22	23
23	27	23	27	23	25	23	25	23	25	23	25	23	24	23	25	23	25	23	25	23	25	23	24
24	28	24	28	24	26	24	26	24	26	24	26	24	25	24	26	24	26	24	26	24	26	24	25
25	29	25	29	25	27	25	27	25	27	25	27	25	26	25	27	25	27	25	27	25	27	25	26
26	30	26	30	26	28	26	28	26	28	26	28	26	27	26	28	26	28	26	28	26	28	26	27
27	31	27	1 (May)	27	29	27	29	27	29	27	29	27	28	27	29	27	29	27	29	27	29	27	28
28	1 (Apr.)	28	2	28	30	28	30	28	30	28	30	28	29	28	30	28	30	28	30	28	30	28	1 (Mar.)
29	2	29	3	29	31 (July)	29	1 (June)	29	31	29	31	29	30	29	31	29	1 (Dec.)	29	31	29	31 (Jan.)	29	2 (Feb.)
30	3			30	1	30	2	30	1 (Aug.)	30	1 (Sep.)	30	1 (Oct.)	30	1 (Nov.)	30	2	30	1	30	1	30	3
31	4			31	2			31	2			31	2	31	2			31	2			31	4

238

PREPARATIONS FOR WHELPING

Preparations for whelping should be made during the last weeks of pregnancy.

First select the whelping area, in a separate room away from any confusion, especially if there are small children or other pets in the house. The area should be warm and well ventilated (but not drafty) and you should be able to draw the drapes or blinds to darken the room if necessary.

Whelping Box

The next essential is a whelping box where the bitch can give birth to her puppies. It can be a simple cardboard carton or a homemade wooden box, and should be large enough for the bitch to lie down or move around comfortably and to accommodate the litter of puppies. The sides should be high enough so that the bitch and her puppies are not bothered by drafts. You will probably be helping your bitch as she whelps; you will need an enclosure that can be cleaned easily and quickly, as there will be a lot of liquid staining.

Illus. 59 shows a cardboard carton that has been converted into a whelping box. All four sides are high enough to keep out drafts but keep in the puppies. One side has been partly cut down to allow the bitch to enter and leave comfortably.

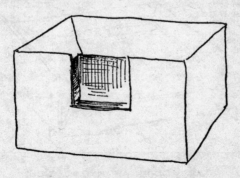

59. CARDBOARD WHELPING BOX

Illus. 60 shows a whelping box which can be constructed of wood. The latched front panel, which can be opened or closed without difficulty, is high enough to restrain the puppies, but lower than the remaining three sides to allow the bitch to enter and leave comfortably.

Illus. 61 shows another type of wooden whelping box. The rail, about 3 inches wide, added around three or four

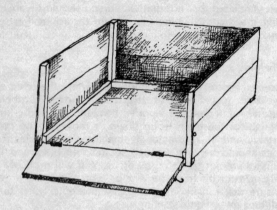

60. WOODEN WHELPING BOX WITH LATCHED PANEL

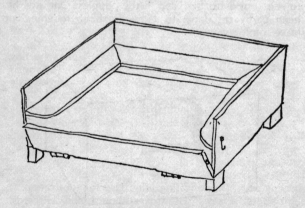

61. WOODEN WHELPING BOX WITH
DROP FRONT AND PIG RAILS

240

sides will allow the puppies to move out of the way when a large or heavy bitch sits or lies down.

The wood used to make the whelping box must be smooth, without any splinters or nails. If you wish to paint or varnish the wood, use a nontoxic finish, as puppies often chew on the sides of their whelping box as they begin to teethe.

The box should be lined with plenty of clean newspapers, which will absorb moisture quickly and can be changed easily. It is not advisable to use sheets or blankets; they become soiled quickly and are difficult to change. Furthermore, newborn puppies can become caught in the folds and smother.

When extra heat is necessary, use a waterproof, chew-resistant kennel heating pad or suspend an infrared lamp over the whelping box, of the type that emits heat but not a lot of bright light, no lower than 2 feet above the bitch's back when she is in the whelping box. For the first 5 days try to maintain a temperature of 85°F, then gradually reduce the temperature over the next few weeks to 75°F to 80°F.

Additional Supplies

A tray or table should be placed near the whelping box with all the supplies that will be needed. These can include:

Rectal thermometer: Use to determine the bitch's temperature before and after whelping.

Cardboard carton: This should be lined with a heating pad or hot-water bottle (either should be well wrapped with soft towels) to temporarily hold each puppy while the dam gives birth to the next.

Towels: Use freshly laundered towels to dry and rub the puppies and to help keep the bitch clean and dry.

Paper towels and cleansing tissues: Use for general cleaning.

Extra newspapers.

Cotton/Q-Tips.

Vaseline® or K-Y lubricating jelly: Use for lubrication.

Blunt-tipped scissors: Use for cutting umbilical cords. Sterilize by placing in boiling water.

Dental floss: Use for tying off umbilical cords.

Antiseptic: Use to swab on umbilical cords.

Flashlight.

Small forceps.

Clock: Use to time the periods between labor and the birth of each puppy.

Pillow: Use for your knees.

Plastic trash bags: Keep two on hand, one for soiled newspapers and paper towels, the other for stained towels and other laundry.

Notebook and pen: Use to record whelping information.

Other items that should be on hand in case of an emergency are:

Baby or food scale (with tray): Use for weighing the puppies.

Premature baby bottle (with preemie nipple) or puppy nursing bottles: Use if it is necessary to hand-feed the puppies.

Bitch's milk substitute such as Esbilac®: This can be purchased from your veterinarian or at most pet shops.

PREWHELPING PREPARATION

Allow the bitch to become accustomed to her whelping box 10 to 12 days before the puppies are due. She should be encouraged to sleep in her box; therefore, make it as cozy as possible for her during the last week. Adding a soft blanket will let her rest more comfortably. She may try to rearrange the blanket several days before the whelping; allow her to do this, but as soon as the first stages of labor begin, remove the blanket and put down newspapers. When whelping is imminent, she will tear and rearrange the newspapers earnestly to prepare her nest.

It is important that hygienic standards be observed for the bitch and her whelping box before, during, and after the birth of the puppies. The whelping box and surrounding areas should be disinfected and kept scrupulously clean at all times.

If the bitch has long hair, it is sanitary to remove the hair from her abdomen a few days before the puppies are due. Trim the hair from around the vulva and breasts with scissors or clippers, *carefully*. Then the pupplies will be able to locate the teats without difficulty and nursing will not be obstructed by clumps of matted hair. If you use scissors, be sure they are blunt-tipped and that you have an assistant steady the bitch as the trimming is being done. If you use clippers, do not trim too closely and irritate the skin. After clipping, the shaved areas should be swabbed with Bactine® or patted with baby lotion to prevent soreness.

As labor approaches, all bitches should be washed gently around the vulva and surrounding areas with a mild antiseptic soap and water. The area should be rinsed and dried thoroughly—and carefully, so that the mother-to-be is not upset.

SIGNS OF LABOR

1. Temperature change: The bitch's normal range of rectal temperature is 100.5°F to 102.5°F (38°C to 39°C). Start checking her temperature several days before the puppies are due. It may fluctuate, depending on time of day. A good indication that puppies will be born within 24 hours is that the bitch's temperature falls and stays below 100°F (37.5°C).

2. Loss of appetite.

3. A watery fluid may be expressed from the nipples.

4. Restlessness and nesting: The bitch will be very restless, panting heavily and tearing up or rearranging the newspapers in her whelping box in a frenzied manner. She may suddenly lie down and be quiet for several minutes, and then begin frantically tearing up newspapers again. She may get in and out of her whelping box frequently.

5. The vulva bcomes swollen, with a mucous discharge from the vagina.

6. The bitch may be very apprehensive. She may stare at her hindquarters or lick her vulva. Panting and trembling will increase and straining will begin.

WHELPING

Most bitches will strain and show contractions at fairly regular intervals. How long the straining will continue varies with the bitch; however, the first puppy should be born within 3 hours after contractions start. If not, call your veterinarian.

As whelping nears, the straining becomes hard and forceful. At this time, some bitches prefer to lie on their sides in the whelping box, while others squat as if they were having a bowel movement. As the contractions increase in strength and frequency, you may see part of a sac (or water bag) of the first fetus emerge from the vulva (Illus. 62). Usually it will be burst by subsequent contractions or by the bitch's continual licking.

Within a few minutes after the water bag has burst, the first puppy will emerge. (*If it is not born within 30 minutes after the water bag bursts, call your veterinarian.*) The head of the puppy appears first, or sometimes the rear end (a breech delivery). The puppy's head and shoulders are the largest parts and require the greatest amount of exertion by the bitch. Once the head is free, the rest of the puppy should be expelled soon after. It should take 1 to 4 minutes for a puppy to be expelled.

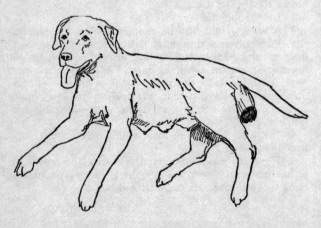

62. WATER BAG

The newborn puppy is enclosed in a slippery membrane with umbilical cord attached. The bitch will turn around and lick or chew away the membrane and sever the puppy's umbilical cord with her teeth. If she appears overwhelmed and does not remove the placental membrane covering the puppy (as sometimes happens with inexperienced bitches), you must do it quickly or the puppy will suffocate. Gently break the membrane open with your finger, then free the head first to allow the puppy to breathe. Open its mouth and clean out any fluids with a gauze dressing. Now clamp the umbilical cord near the center with a small forceps or sterile umbilical cord clamp. Tie the cord firmly with dental floss about an inch or 2 from the puppy's body, being careful not to pull the stomach wall. Then cut the umbilical cord (Illus. 63), with sterilized blunt-tipped scissors (these should have been placed in boiling water beforehand, then wiped with alcohol). After the cord is cut, remove the forceps or umbilical cord clamp and swab the end with tincture of merthiolate or other liquid antiseptic.

Dry the puppy briskly with a small terry towel and place it next to its mother. She will begin to lick the puppy forcefully and you may hear it gasp or cry. Often, the bitch will direct the puppy toward her nipples, or it will nose around and find her breasts without help and begin

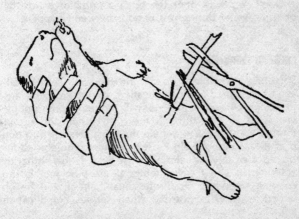

63. TYING AND CUTTING THE UMBILICAL CORD

245

to nurse. If the puppy does not start to nurse within a short time, try expressing a little milk from one of the nipples, then put the puppy's mouth to it.

In 15 to 60 minutes after the birth of the first puppy, the bitch will begin straining again to deliver the second, repeating the same steps—delivery of the fetus, breaking the placental membrane, severing the umbilical cord, drying the puppy—until the entire litter is born.

If the bitch is straining or moving about a great deal, separate the newborn puppies from her while she gives birth to the rest. Place the puppies in a small cardboard container (prepared in advance by lining the bottom with a heating pad or hot-water bottle and covering the pad or bottle with a soft terry towel). Place the box close to the bitch where she can see her puppies, as she will be greatly disturbed if they are out of sight.

Normally the afterbirth is expelled with or just after a puppy is born or just before the next puppy is born. There is one afterbirth for each puppy: be careful to count the afterbirths to be sure they have all been expelled from the uterus, as a retained placenta can cause serious problems. The bitch will try to eat the afterbirth once a puppy is delivered. It is not necessary, however, to permit her to eat every one of them, which can cause diarrhea and vomiting. Allowing her to eat one or two afterbirths will be sufficient.

Don't forget to offer the bitch a drink of warm milk or some water during rest periods between puppies.

Difficult Deliveries

Sometimes whelpings do not proceed as systematically as just described and complications occur. Problems arise in abnormal (and some normal) presentations, puppies too large to pass through the birth canal, and uterine inertia. You may have to help the bitch give birth to puppies if she cannot help herself. Serious problems should be reported to your veterinarian at once. Don't bother the veterinarian about trivial things if the whelping is proceeding smoothly, but professional help should be obtained as soon as possible when *serious* complications arise.

If the head or rear end passes out and the bitch has

difficulty expelling the rest of the puppy, scrub your hands (*fingernails, especially*) and spread K-Y lubricating jelly or Vaseline® around the vulva and as much of the exposed puppy as you can. Be careful not to push the puppy back up into the birth canal or to damage the delicate tissue.

After lubrication, try to keep the bitch in a standing position, rather than a crouching position as if she were attempting to have a bowel movement. Grasp the exposed part carefully with a gauze dressing, terry fingertip towel, or clean handkerchief; during the next contraction, gently pull with an outward and downward motion. Repeat this action with each contraction until the puppy is expelled. *Do not try to pull the puppy out by force.* If the puppy is still not expelled in a short time, call your veterinarian immediately.

Difficult birth also may be caused by puppies too large to pass through the birth canal or uterine inertia, a condition where the uterus fails to contract adequately and the bitch cannot expel her puppies. It can be the result of prolonged straining for 2 to 3 hours with no puppies being born (old, overweight, under-exercised bitches are prone to this) or it can be an inherited trait where the contractions will never be strong enough to expel the puppies. Other causes include trauma or overexcitement during delivery, perhaps caused by noisy children, other pets, or strangers being permitted to watch the delivery or by the bitch not feeling secure in her whelping quarters. Uterine inertia must be dealt with by a veterinarian at once. The problem can be corrected by one of the following:

1. Internal manipulations and use of forceps by the veterinarian to deliver the puppies. *An inexperienced person should never attempt to manually manipulate a puppy in the birth canal*
2. Injection of a hormone to stimulate or renew uterine contractions
3. Removing the puppies by cesarean section

Weak and Lifeless Puppies

Most puppies are born healthy, but occasionally one will appear to be weak or lifeless, with bluish skin, shallow, uneven, or no breathing. Even if a puppy looks lifeless, you may be able to revive it by immediately performing the following steps:

1. Clear the mouth, nose, and chest of fluids.
   a. Wrap a gauze dressing around your fingertip. Open the puppy's mouth, pull its tongue forward, and swab away any fluids.
   b. Hold the puppy with its head downward securely in the palms of your hands. Use your fingers to maintain its head and spine in a straight line (Illus. 64).

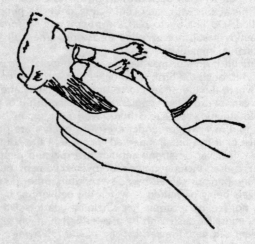

64. DOWNWARD SWING HOLD

   c. Lift your arms above your head and swing the puppy downward between your legs (Illus. 65). Repeat several times. The force of the swing will help to drain fluids from the puppy's chest, throat, and nose.
2. Hold the puppy in a warm towel and rub it briskly to stimulate circulation and breathing. If the brisk rubbing makes the hair fall out, the puppy has been dead for a while.
3. Sometimes a *drop* of brandy on the tongue will make the puppy gasp and begin breathing.

4. If you do not get a response from swinging and rubbing the puppy briskly, try giving artificial respiration. Carefully and gently depress the chest with your thumb and index finger for about 2 seconds, then release the

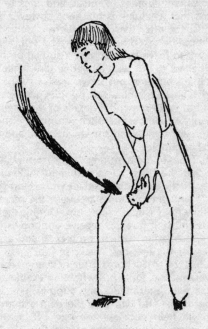

65. DOWNWARD SWING

pressure for about 2 seconds. You can also try mouth-to-nose resuscitation by placing your mouth over the puppy's muzzle and blowing gently into the nostrils for 2 seconds, then removing your mouth for 2 seconds to permit the air to be expelled from the lungs. *Air must be blown gently into the nostrils to avoid damaging the puppy's lungs.* Either method should be tried for several minutes.

5. If the puppy begins to breathe normally and its skin becomes a pinkish color, return it to its dam.

POSTWHELPING CARE

How can you tell when all of the puppies have been born? When the bitch relaxes and stops panting and trembling, allows her puppies to nurse, and tries to rest, you can assume that whelping is finished; however, puppies have been born after these signs were observed.

The bitch should be taken out to relieve herself, though she will not want to leave her puppies. You will probably have to force her to go out with someone else while you clean the whelping box and put down fresh newspapers. This is a good time to examine the puppies for possible deformities and to write down the details of the whelping in your notebook. As soon as the bitch returns, she should be offered some warm milk and soft, bland food and then left alone with her puppies.

Check from time to time during the first few hours after delivery that the bitch has a sufficient milk supply for the puppies. If she does not, contact your veterinarian immediately. The nursing period starts with the secretion of a watery-milky fluid called colostrum. During the first 24 hours of life, nursing puppies receive antibodies from their mother's colostrum which protect them against certain diseases for the first few weeks of life.

During the first 24 to 36 hours after delivery, take the bitch to the veterinarian for a postwhelping examination. The veterinarian will determine if any puppies have been retained in the uterus and will give the dam a hormone injection that will help decrease the size of the uterus and expel any retained puppies or afterbirths. The hormone also helps let down the bitch's milk. It is important that the mother be examined soon after delivery, since a retained puppy or afterbirth can cause an infection and make her seriously ill.

The bitch's bowel movements may be soft and dark for a day or two after whelping, especially if she has eaten several afterbirths. This is normal, but the stools should return to their original color and consistency within a few days. A blood-tinged discharge for 7 to 10 days after delivery is normal; it should decrease gradually, become clear, and then stop altogether. In case of a heavy, foul-smelling discharge or elevated temperature, inform your veterinarian as soon as possible.

For the first day or 2 after whelping feed the bitch milk and meat broths along with soft, bland foods. Feed her as much and as often as she wishes. By the third day she can resume her regular diet; this should be supplemented with high-protein foods, such as cooked eggs, cottage cheese, liver and other meats, and milk. If milk causes loose bowel movements, discontinue it in favor of other high-protein foods. Nursing a litter of puppies places a heavy nutritional demand on the bitch. If you are concerned about what she should eat, find out from your veterinarian what kinds of high-quality food and vitamin-mineral supplements are necessary.

Danger Signs

Call your veterinarian if one or more of these signs of serious problems appears:

1. Pregnancy lasting longer than 68 days
2. Forceful straining for longer than 2 to 3 hours
3. Agonized screaming by the bitch
4. Dark greenish foul-smelling discharge
5. Excessive bleeding
6. Contractions weakening or stopping after 1 or 2 puppies
7. Head, rear, or other part of a puppy stuck in the vulva
8. Prolonged appearance and disappearance of a bubble at the vulva
9. Elevated rectal temperature of bitch after delivery
10. Restless, whimpering puppies
11. Absence of the bitch's milk
12. Increased restlessness of the mother after whelping, particularly trembling and spasms of the head and legs
13. Bitch has hard, enlarged, discolored breasts
14. The bitch secretes off-color milk or other fluids
15. Prolonged dark red, foul-smelling vaginal discharge (with or without pus)

POSTWHELPING COMPLICATIONS

Agalactia

Agalactia is absence or failure of secretion of the bitch's milk. It can be inherited, or caused by an imbalance of hormones or nervousness. It is relatively common, especially in young bitches of certain breeds.

During the first 24 hours, the litter should be watched carefully to see that they are getting enough nourishment. Contented puppies are quiet and sleep most of the time between nursings. Puppies that are not receiving nourishment are restless. They crawl erratically around the litter box and cry and whimper a great deal because they are hungry. The combination of stress and lack of food can cause the puppies to weaken rapidly and become dehydrated. To test for dehydration, pinch a fold of skin on the back of a puppy's neck. It should go back into position immediately: if it is slow to go back into place or remains pinched together, the puppy is dehydrated.

If you notice symptoms of hunger in the newborn puppies, consult your veterinarian immediately. The mother can be given an injection of hormones to stimulate the flow of milk. This tends to be effective only when the condition is observed early, and is one important reason why the bitch should receive a postwhelping examination by a veterinarian 24 to 36 hours after delivery. The injection usually will be effective within 24 hours, but until the time milk is flowing, the puppies will have to be hand-fed. (See "Puppies: Orphan Puppies.") If injections to stimulate milk flow are ineffective, the puppies will have to be hand-fed until they can eat by themselves.

Eclampsia

Eclampsia (milk fever) can occur anytime during the first 4 weeks after the puppies are born, and also during the last 2 weeks of pregnancy. The exact cause is unknown, but in eclampsia the blood calcium level drops below normal. The condition usually occurs in small or medium-sized bitches, especially those with large litters and ample quantities of milk.

Eclampsia is a serious emergency that requires immediate veterinary treatment. There is no way to prevent eclampsia, but try to become familiar with the symptoms and watch for their appearance during the nursing period. The onset of eclampsia is rapid and the bitch can die in 12 to 24 hours if untreated.

Symptoms of Eclampsia

* Bitch becomes nervous and excited.
* Breathing may be shallow and rapid at first; then labored as the condition progresses.
* Increased restlessness: bitch may pace about or get in and out of her whelping box constantly.
* Staggering gait.
* Profuse salivation.
* Trembling and spasms, especially of the head and legs. Eventually, the bitch may lie on her side and move her legs in jerky motions.
* High rectal temperature.
* Collapse.
* Convulsions (advanced stage).

Emergency Action for Eclampsia

Get the bitch immediately to a veterinarian for intravenous injections of calcium gluconate and other medical treatment. Don't delay. A major cause of death in eclampsia is brain damage from high temperature. If your bitch is having seizures and you cannot reach a veterinarian quickly, take her rectal temperature frequently. If it goes above 103°F (39.5°C), activate an instant cold pack and place it on the back of the neck, or wrap the bitch in cold towels to help lower her temperature. Maintaining the temperature near 102°F (39°C) may mean the difference between life and death. After the bitch has been treated, the puppies may be allowed limited nursing at most; they will have to be fed a commercially made bitch's milk substitute to assure their survival. Puppies old enough to eat by themselves should be weaned. When eclampsia is treated promptly, most bitches recover quickly with no complications.

Excess Milk—Mastitis

Mastitis is an inflammation of the mammary glands caused by an infection in the bitch. An overabundance of milk can cause the bitch's teats to become swollen and inflamed. Because the area is so painful, she often refuses to let the puppies nurse from the affected breasts. A lumpy, discolored, or enlarged breast or breasts may indicate mastitis. Because the condition develops quickly, it is suggested that the bitch's breasts be examined every day for the symptoms listed below.

Symptoms of Excess Milk—Mastitis

• One or more breasts especially the two lower breasts, may appear lumpy and swollen.
• Reddish purple discoloration of the affected breasts.
• Affected breasts feel hot and hard to the touch.
• Decreased appetite.
• Unwillingness to nurse puppies.
• Constipation.
• Diarrhea.
• High rectal temperature—often over 104°F (40°C).
• Off-color milk (sometimes brownish or bloodstained). Squeeze a small quantity of milk from an affected breast on a white facial tissue or paper towel. Then extract several drops of milk from an unaffected breast and compare color and uniformity. If there is a difference, the bitch may have mastitis.

Emergency Action for Excess Milk—Mastitis

1. For inflammation and swelling *with no temperature elevation,* apply moist warm compresses to the affected breast(s) for 30 minutes every 2 hours. As the breast softens from the warm compresses, gently squeeze the teat and try to withdraw as much milk as possible. Relief is generally obtained after several treatments.
2. If the breasts still remain hard and discolored and the rectal temperature is elevated to 103°F to 104°F (39.5°C to 40°C), this indicates infection. *If prompt treatment is not begun, the breasts may become abscessed.*
3. Take the bitch to a veterinarian immediately. Remove

the puppies from nursing: if they consume their mother's infected milk, they will become seriously ill. They should be fed a commercially made bitch's milk substitute to help assure their survival (see "Puppies: Orphan Puppies") until the veterinarian determines that the bitch can resume nursing.

Metritis

Metritis is an inflammation of the uterus that can be caused by difficult labor; retained afterbirth, fetal membranes, or a dead fetus; unclean whelping quarters; manual internal manipulations; or incorrect use of instruments. Either bacteria enter the uterus or an infection arises from decomposing membranes retained in the uterus.

Symptoms of Metritis

- Listlessness.
- Bitch may be uninterested in her puppies.
- Loss of appetite.
- Excessive thirst.
- Dark red, foul-smelling vaginal discharge.
- High rectal temperature.
- If not treated, the discharge becomes very dark and may contain pus. The uterus becomes enlarged and tender and the bitch experiences great pain when the abdomen is touched.

Emergency Action for Metritis

1. Take the bitch to a veterinarian for immediate treatment. If ignored, metritis can be fatal.
2. Remove the puppies from nursing. The dam's milk may be toxic and the puppies may have to be fed a commercially made substitute for bitch's milk.

Loss of Hair

Often after whelping and nursing a litter of puppies, the bitch's coat may look dry and lifeless or begin to fall out. This is often the result of an inadequate diet, as nursing places a heavy nutritional burden on the dam. When the diet is adequate and the puppies have been weaned, the hair will gradually return to normal.

PUPPIES

Weighing Puppies

Each puppy should be weighed at birth, at 12 hours, at 24 hours, and daily for at least 10 days. Use a platform food scale (with weighing tray) to weigh newborn puppies: it accurately measures ounces as well as pounds. Normal puppies should:

1. Gain weight steadily from the beginning of nursing; or lose less than 10% of their birth weight during the first 48 hours, then start to gain steadily
2. Double their birth weight by age 10 to 12 days

Characteristics of Normal Young Puppy

We assume the litter box is maintained at 85°F (29.4C°).

Rectal temperature: 94°F to 99°F (34.5°C to 37.2°C)
Respiration: 20 to 30 breaths per minute
Heart rate: Approximately 200 beats per minute
Sucking instinct: Strong and vigorous
Mucous membranes: Bright reddish pink
Coat: Dry and smooth
Body: Warm to the touch
Crying: Little or none
Frequently relaxes on its side with legs extended. Presence of occasional muscle twitching
Puppy has no trouble moving toward or finding its dam
Stimulation: Good reflexes. Stroking the back often stimulates vigorous activity

Characteristics of Sick Young Puppy

We assume the litter box is maintained at 85°F (29.4C°).

These are all danger signs:

Incessant crying and restlessness. Sick puppies will not stay with their mother: they may go off by themselves or crawl erratically around the litter box

Failure to gain in weight or size
Coat: May feel harsh and damp
Sucking instinct: Weak or absent
Slow and shallow respiration and heart rate
Yellow diarrhea
Body: Feels cold and clammy to the touch
Mucous membranes: Pale or bluish
Low rectal temperature
When turned on its back, the puppy will not roll over immediately on its stomach
Poor reflexes: Will not move toward its mother
Puppy will be bloated
Dehydration: Pinch a fold of skin on the back of the neck. It should go back into position immediately. If the skin is slow to go back into place or remains pinched together, the puppy has lost considerable fluids and is dehydrated

AVERAGE RECTAL TEMPERATURES FOR NORMAL PUPPIES

Week	°F	°C
1–2	95–99	35–37.2
2–4	97–101	36.1–38.3

TEMPERATURE REQUIREMENTS OF THE WHELPING/NURSING AREA

Week	°F	°C
1st	85	29.5
2nd	80	27
3rd	75	24
4th+	70	21.5

AVERAGE TIMETABLE FOR NORMAL PUPPIES

Event	Time After Birth (days)
Crawling	0 (birth)
Umbilical cord dries and falls off	2–3
Body weight should double	10–12

Event	Time After Birth (days)
Eyes open (unless litter was premature)	10–14
Ears open (unless litter was premature)	15–17
Standing upright and walking	19–21
Appearance of canine teeth	21
Owner recognition	24–28
Appearance of premolars	28
Running	28
Weaning	28–42

Early Care

During the first 3 weeks the bitch should be totally devoted to caring for her puppies. If she is relaxed and the puppies are contented and sleep soundly between meals, you can be reasonably sure that they are nursing properly; however, keep watch on the mother and puppies to be sure no nursing problems are developing.

If a puppy refuses to nurse or has difficulty nursing, you may have to teach it how to suck by holding it at the bitch's breast and squeezing some of her milk into its mouth. Once a puppy gets a taste of the milk, it will generally begin to nurse. If the puppy still refuses to nurse or is weak, or if the bitch does not have an adequate supply of milk, you will have to hand-feed a commercially made bitch's milk substitute. (See: "Puppies: Hand-Feeding Puppies.")

If the litter is small in number, notice if the puppies are nursing from all of the breasts. If they are not, place them on different breasts during a 24-hour period, especially the teats that are most filled with milk. Otherwise some of the breasts (especially the two lower ones) may become inflamed and caked with milk. Then when the puppies attempt to nurse on a swollen breast, the bitch may be in such pain that she will not permit them to. The caked breast will have to be hand-milked until relief is obtained. (See "Postwhelping Complications: Excess Milk —Mastitis.")

For a litter that is large in number, check that there are enough teats for the puppies. Try to put the weaker or smaller puppies to the breasts first for feeding, as they often get pushed away by the larger puppies; but remember that while you want to provide an adequate supply of milk to encourage the weaker puppies to grow, you are not trying to starve the larger puppies or suppress their development. Supplemental feeding of a bitch's milk substitute may be necessary when there are many puppies, especially if they are not growing.

Dewclaws should be removed and tails docked (when required in your breed) by a veterinarian when the puppies are 3 to 4 days old. About the 4th day, the sharp points of the puppies' nails should be trimmed. The ends of the nails grow sharp quickly and should be trimmed weekly thereafter; if they are allowed to grow long, they can scratch the bitch's teats as the puppies nurse. Each puppy's rear end should be checked daily. Generally the bitch will keep her puppies licked clean, but if she does not, the puppies' anal areas can become clogged. If this happens, moisten a cotton ball with warm water and gently clean the rectal area. Dry thoroughly and apply a little Vaseline® if the area is irritated.

The bitch should be checked daily to see that her abdominal and rectal areas are clean, that no breasts are caked with milk or discolored, and that the puppies are not scratching her teats. Throughout the nursing period the whelping box, the bedding, and the surrounding areas should be kept scrupulously clean.

Orphan Puppies

Warmth is essential to a newborn puppy. Chilling is the greatest danger to young puppies, whose abilities to control body temperatures are not completely developed. Puppies that have lost their mother or have been isolated from their mother to keep them from nursing on her should be maintained in a warm, dry, draft-free environment. The whelping-box temperature should be carefully maintained at the levels suggested in the table "Temperature Requirements of the Whelping/Nursing Area" (p. 257). The best way to assure an even, warm temperature is to use an overhead infrared lamp or heating pad. If the pad is not waterproof, it should be covered with some type of impermeable material and then sealed in a towel or other soft fabric. Keep the heating pad set on "low" and be sure the seal is secure enough to prevent a puppy from crawling between the towel (or soft fabric) and the pad. Cover only half of the bottom of the litter box with the heating pad so that the puppies can get near the heat when they are cold or get away from it when they are hot. Too much heat is as dangerous as chilling: it can cause dehydration. If necessary, keep a thermometer in the litter box so you can be sure the temperature is correct.

The puppies should be rubbed with a moistened washcloth occasionally, and dried thoroughly to keep them clean. If the skin appears dry and flaky, rub a little baby oil into it to help restore moisture.

When puppies cannot nurse at their mother's breasts, they will try to suck at each other's tail, feet, ears, or genitals to satisfy the sucking instinct. Bottle feeding may satisfy the puppies' urge to suck; but should you notice the puppies beginning to nurse on their littermates, you may have to put them in separate sections of the litter box for the first few weeks to prevent injury. Don't disturb the puppies except for feeding and cleaning. Newborn puppies are like newborn babies: for the first few weeks they should be eating or sleeping. If the puppies have not nursed and received the mother's colostrum (the watery-milky secretion from the breasts immediately after delivery from which protective substances pass from the bitch's body to her puppies), check with your veterinarian as soon as possible to determine when the puppies will receive temporary immunization.

Hand-Feeding Puppies

The following are some of the reasons why you may have to handfeed a litter of puppies:

1. Orphan puppies
2. Absence of the bitch's milk (agalactia)
3. Mastitis infection
4. Eclampsia
5. Supplemental feeding of puppies too weak to nurse or too small to compete with their littermates
6. Supplemental feeding of a litter with many puppies
7. Mother's refusal to nurse one or more puppies

In addition, if the puppies were delivered by cesarean section, hand feeding may be necessary during the first few days of life.

What to Feed

There are several commercially prepared powder or liquid substitutes for bitch's milk, such as Esbilac® and Orphalac®, which can be obtained at most pet stores or from your veterinarian. Cow's milk and human baby formulas are not suitable for puppies because they do not provide the same nutritional balance that is contained in the bitch's milk. It is wise to keep a can of bitch's milk substitute on hand for emergencies.

Should you not have a commercially prepared bitch's milk substitute on hand, either of the following emergency formulas can be used temporarily:

FORMULA #1

3 parts canned evaporated milk
1 part boiled water (cooled to room temperature)
1/4 teaspoon Dicalcium Phosphate for each cup of evaporated milk used (available at most pharmacies and health food or certain pet stores)

FORMULA #2

1 cup canned evaporated milk
1 cup boiling water (cooled to room temperature)
1 egg yolk
1 tablespoon Karo syrup (light or dark)
1 teaspoon limewater

Both formulas should be mixed and stored in the refrigerator. At feeding time, the formula should be mixed well and an amount sufficient for a feeding of the entire litter should be removed and warmed.

How Much to Feed

In *The Collins Guide to Dog Nutrition*, Dr. Donald R. Collins recommends:

261

If their formula resembles bitch's milk closely enough, newborn puppies of small and medium-size breeds do not need to be fed more than four times daily. For larger breeds, this number may need to be increased to six. To determine the daily quantity to feed each puppy, the following calorie intakes for preweaning puppies should be used:

weeks of age	required calories per pound of body weight	required calories per ounce of body weight
1st	60	3.7
2nd	70	4.4
3d	80–90	5.0–5.6
4th	90+	5.6+

Using these figures with a formula of proper content, the total daily quantity required will divide into four to six equal feedings that will leave the puppy with a moderately distended stomach following each feeding. The exact quantity to be fed must always be left to the discretion of the person feeding the puppy. Common sense is still one of the most important aspects of successfully raising infant pups. Just remember, *it is better to underfeed them than to overfeed*. Start with the figure given, as a guide to estimate the quantity needed, then let the puppy tell you how much it really needs.

For example, a puppy weighing 1 pound requires 60 calories per day; one weighing 10 ounces requires $37\frac{1}{2}$ calories per day. The calorie content of most commercially prepared bitch's milk substitutes is listed on the label, making the table above easy to follow. If the calorie content is not listed, following the manufacturer's directions for feeding.

Dr. Collins explains that there are several ways to determine if a puppy is getting too much or too little food. Crying, a common sign can be inaccurate because puppies not only cry when they are hungry but also when they are cold, hot, or otherwise disturbed. He states that a puppy's systemic reactions are good indicators of whether it is eating enough and that each time a puppy is fed, it should have a bowel movement and urinate. Dr. Collins adds:

The character and amount of a pup's feces and urine are important clues that tell you how well you are doing as its mother. A puppy's stool should be formed as it is expelled, but its consistency should be soft and pasty. Its color will depend to some extent on what you are feeding the pup. But in every case, it should range from a pale tan to a mahogany brown. The inside of the stool may be yellow-brown in many cases, but this is not objectionable. Stools that are green, bluish white, or clear signal trouble. Even tan or brownish stools that are watery, lumpy, hard, or curdled may indicate something is wrong. Whenever either off-color or off-form stools occur, stop feeding immediately and skip the next feeding entirely. Begin the following feeding with a formula that has been diluted one-half with boiling water. Continue to feed the same quantity as you did of the undiluted food. If this fails to produce an improvement in the stool, cut the quantity you are feeding by 25 percent at each feeding. If the stools continue to be off-color or off-form, call your veterinarian.

A puppy's urination is an indicator of its water balance. The quantity should be about the same each time the puppy urinates. It might be pale yellow to almost clear, but should never be deep yellow or orange. It should always be like water and never like syrup. It should smell like urine. Urine that is scanty, dark in color, or syrupy indicates that the pup is not receiving enough water. Additional water should be supplied, either added to the formula or fed separately. If the urine seems excessive in amount, unduly clear, or thin, the water concentration of the formula should be reexamined to make certain that too much water is not being given. If urine production stops altogether for longer than four feedings, take the puppy to a veterinarian promptly.

Feeding Procedures

The most common method of hand-feeding young puppies is to use a nursing bottle and nipple. You will need small animal-nursing bottles designed for young puppies. These are especially recommended for nursing small breeds. For larger breeds (or in case puppy nursing bottles are not available), nursing bottles and anticolic nipples designed for premature human babies are suggested.

Use separate bottles for each puppy if possible, and sterilize the bottles (and their nipples) before feeding. If you use a commercially prepared bitch's milk substitute, follow the manufacturer's mixing and feeding directions carefully. The formula should be fed at room temperature or slightly warmer. Test the nipple before feeding to be sure the milk will flow properly. The formula should drop slowly from the opening as the bottle is held upside down; if it does not, the hole should be enlarged.

Step-by-Step Instructions for Hand Feeding

1. The best way to feed a puppy is to place it on its stomach on a warm, folded terry towel. The thickness of the towel will give the puppy a surface to press against, as it would against the bitch's teats if it were nursing naturally.

2. Open the mouth and before inserting the nipple, use your finger to determine if the puppy's tongue is down and forward. Newborn puppies have tongues as thin as tissue paper: do not force the nipple into the mouth if the tongue is sticking to the roof.

3. Once the tongue is in place, slide the nipple into the mouth as you remove your finger. To encourage the puppy to start nursing, squeeze a drop of milk onto the tip of the nipple before you insert it. *Do not, however, squeeze milk from the nipple when it is in the puppy's mouth*.

4. Hold the bottle upward (not too high) in a position that does not allow the entry of too much air, which may cause colic.

5. Usually, normal hungry puppies will suck energetically after tasting the milk.

6. If a puppy is too weak to be fed on its stomach, hold it upright in your hand (Illus. 66). *Do not feed a puppy on its back and do not use an eyedropper to give formula to the puppy; either procedure can allow the puppy to inhale milk into its lungs.*

7. Don't allow the puppy to nurse too quickly. If milk bubbles from the nose or mouth the formula is being consumed too quickly.

8. Should the puppy choke or gag, immediately take the bottle out of its mouth and

    a. Hold the puppy with its head downward *securely* in the palms of your hands. Use your fingers to maintain its head and spine in a straight line.

    b. Lift your arms above your head and swing the puppy downward between your legs. Repeat this movement several times to help drain the milk from the puppy's trachea and throat. (See Illus. 64, 65.)

9. After each feeding, burp the puppy by holding it upright in your hand and patting or stroking its back.

10. Orphan puppies or those not cared for by their mothers require additional care. When the bitch licks her puppies after feeding, she stimulates the processes of urination and defecation. If the mother is not available after each feeding, you will have to stimulate the pup-

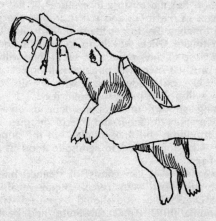

66. BOTTLE FEEDING OF WEAK PUPPY

pies to get rid of their wastes by moistening a cotton ball with warm water and rubbing over the rectal and abdominal areas. This artificial stimulation will be necessary for the first 7 to 10 days of the puppies lives; afterward they become self-regulating.

11. Weigh each puppy carefully every day, and using Dr. Collins's table as a guideline, increase the food intake along with the increase in body weight.

12. Wean the puppies as soon as possible.

Another method of hand-feeding puppies is to pass a catheter or small feeding tube over the tongue and into the puppy's stomach. Before attempting this feeding method, contact your veterinarian for the correct equipment and a demonstration of the precise technique of inserting the tube.

WHEN TO BEGIN WEANING

Orphan puppies or those not being nursed by their mothers should be introduced to a soupy form of solid food at about 2 weeks of age. Use jars of human baby food containing meat, or Prescription Diet® i/d® and add enough formula (bitch's milk substitute) to make a syrupy consistency. Put the mixture in a saucer or flat dish, dip your finger in the food, and rub it around the puppies' lips and tongues. Try to get the puppies to lick the food off your finger. Once they learn to lick the food, hold the dish close to their mouths to see if they will lick the mixture on their own. The puppies will not eat much at this early age, but gradually, and with a little help from you they will accept more semisolid food.

Weaning age for normal puppies depends on a number of considerations (number and size of puppies, mother's general condition and milk supply), but the puppies can in general be introduced to semisolid food at about 3 weeks of age.

The weaning diet can consist of strained baby meat, instant high-protein baby cereal, puppy meal, or Prescription Diet®. The food should be mixed with equal parts formula (bitch's milk substitute) and beaten well with a fork or eggbeater or in a blender.

Before you first offer semisolid food, keep the bitch away from her puppies for a short time to be sure they are hungry. The mixture should be put in a flat dish or pie tin and taken to the whelping box. You will have to teach the puppies how to lick by spreading some of the food on their lips and tongue. Once a hungry puppy licks the food on its lips or from your fingers, put the pan down in the whelping box. Some puppies may start to lap the food immediately, while others will try to walk into the pan or sit in it! Just maintain your patience and sense of humor for a short time because, eventually, all the puppies will learn to eat. Watch, though, to be sure that smaller, weaker puppies are not being pushed away from the food by those larger, stronger ones. The food pans should be scrubbed thoroughly between feedings and a pan of water should be available after the puppies are 3 weeks of age.

Once they become accustomed to eating the soupy mixture, the amount of formula should be gradually decreased over the next 2 weeks until the puppies are eating solid food. While the puppies are still feeding from their mother as well, give three meals a day. Sometimes at weaning the mother may regurgitate partly digested food for her puppies. This is a normal occurrence, believed to be a throwback to times when wild dogs would regurgitate food to sustain their puppies.

By the time the puppies are 5 weeks old, most of their baby teeth are in and the mother becomes hesitant to nurse as it becomes increasingly uncomfortable. As you gradually increase the amount of solid food given to the puppies, gradually reduce the bitch's food intake and limit the amount of nursing time with the puppies. By 6 to 7 weeks the puppies should be weaned, eating three meals a day. Fresh drinking water should be available at all times. By this time also, the bitch's food intake should be down to the level that existed before pregnancy. The reduced food intake will help naturally decrease her milk production; however, if it does not dry up sufficiently and the bitch is suffering, consult your veterinarian.

PUPPY VACCINATIONS

Information about vaccination against distemper, hepatitis, leptospirosis, and canine parainfluenza is in section IV, but we will mention here that puppies usually receive their first immunization shots when they are 7 to 8 weeks of age and then have one or two more shots at 2-week intervals.

PUPPY SOCIALIZATION

Developing a puppy's temperament is as important as developing a strong, healthy body. Part of being a responsible dog breeder or owner involves making a puppy more adaptable to today's life through correct socialization during the critical period when the puppy's personality is being formed.

Socialization can be defined as the way in which a dog develops a relationship with its mother, littermates, other animals, and humans.

A dog should be friendly to other dogs as well as motivated by and oriented toward humans. A puppy needs socialization with its mother, its littermates, and humans. If it does not get these at the proper time, the puppy may never reach its mental or social potential and may exhibit temperament problems. Puppies and children possess the same emotional centers and, in principle, go through the same developmental periods. It is not surprising therefore, that many of the behavior problems observed in dogs have been recorded by child psychiatrists.

Some years ago a project directed by Drs. J. Paul Scott and John Fuller was undertaken at the Animal Behavior Laboratory of the Jackson Memorial Laboratory, Bar Harbor, Maine, to determine the critical periods in a puppy's life. The results were so significant that the Guide Dogs Foundation adopted them for raising puppies to be guide dogs for the blind.

The first critical period is the first 20 days of a puppy's

life. It involves survival. The puppy's reflexes are concerned mainly with movement towards its mother as she feeds, cleans, and keeps the puppy warm in the nest. It has been determined through scientific tests that puppies are not capable of learning anything during the first critical period.

The second critical period begins on the 21st day, when the senses begin to function and the puppy reacts to its environment and its littermates. During this period, which lasts through the 28th day of the puppy's life, it needs to be with its mother and littermates. Tail wagging, playing, barking, and play fighting (complete with tiny growls) begin. Since the dog is a pack animal, you should notice the beginnings of a social hierarchy, in which a dominant puppy will emerge, with the others deferring to it. The rest of the puppies will quickly find their places in the litter's pecking order. During this week, it is important that the puppy not be separated from its mother or littermates; otherwise, it may never learn to fully adjust to other dogs.

The third critical period begins immediately after the second, and lasts from the 5th through the 7th week. Now the puppy recognizes people and responds to voices. In addition to mother/littermate socialization, it needs daily periods of human socialization. You should handle the puppy, pet it, give it lots of affection, and play with it. If a puppy does not receive the required human socialization at this time, it may be unfriendly or asocial with people.

The best time to take the puppy away from its mother and littermates and place it in a new home is between 6 to 8 weeks. Now the puppy can accept its new owner as "pack" leader and be more trainable. When a puppy is left with its mother and littermates after 8 weeks of age, it becomes too dog-oriented and difficult to train.

The next critical period is when the puppy is 8 to 12 weeks old. From 8 to 9 weeks learning becomes more fixed, but because an anxiety period develops, this can be a sensitive time. Simple commands ("Sit," "Stay," "Come"), housebreaking, and lead training can begin at 8 weeks when a puppy is most sensitive to *mild* discipline; but training should be started gently with plenty of praise given as a reward. Do not make the training sessions too long. Very young puppies are highly motivated by and responsive to their owners, but like babies, they have short periods of concentration. Although intelligence develops rapidly in a puppy, early training should be started on a fun basis. Don't punish a puppy severely at this age or you can destroy its bond with humans.

Supervised play with children can begin, but do not allow a child to scare or abuse a puppy, on purpose or unintentionally. If you want to develop every potential of the new puppy, experiences away from home are as important as human socialization now. Take the puppy out for short walks, rides in the car, or short errands (after it has been inoculated, of course!) where it can meet other people. Such activities will not frighten a puppy now if they are accompanied by lots of encouragement, praise, and love.

To understand more about the critical periods in a puppy's life and the effects of improper socialization on later development, we recommend that every dog owner read *Understanding Your Dog* by Dr. Michael W. Fox and *The New Knowledge of Dog Behavior* by Clarence J. Pfaffenberger. (See "For Additional Reading: Behavior and Training" at the end of the book.) By knowing the basics of proper socialization, you can help to provide the best environment for a dog's potential to be developed and to prevent behavioral problems in future litters.

Section IV

HEALTH CARE

VITAL STATISTICS AND MEDICAL RECORD OF

_____
(Dog's Call Name)

Registered Name _____
                        (If purebred)

Breed _____

Birth Date _____

Sex _____

Registration No. _____
                        (If registered with AKC, etc.)

Color and Markings _____

Distinguishing Features _____

Ears _____Eyes _____

Coat _____

Sire (Father) _____

Dam (Mother) _____

Date Acquired _____From Whom _____

Address _____

License Tag No. _____

Rabies Tag No. _____

Veterinarian _____

Hospital Address _____

IMMUNIZATION AND BOOSTER SHOT RECORD

	Date	Date	Date	Date	Date	Date
Canine distemper						
Canine hepatitis						
Canine leptospirosis						
Parainfluenza vaccine						
Rabies						

GENERAL HEALTH

	Date	Date	Date	Date
Physical examination				
Worming (record date, and type of worm)				
Heartworm check				
Medical problem or chronic condition				
Major illness				
Allergy				
Surgery or hospitalization				
Heat period				

Date of spaying or neutering _____

Veterinarian:

Alternate veterinarian:

Animal emergency clinic:

Local Poison Control Center:

Drugstore:

ASPCA or Humane Society:

Police:

Other:

Keep a clear color snapshot of a sideview of your dog for identification purposes in case your pet is lost or stolen. If your dog's sides have different markings, keep a color snapshot of each side.

A BRIEF GUIDE TO DOG OWNERSHIP

Choose a dog that will best suit your life-style. Dog ownership involves certain responsibilities; here are some suggestions that may help decide the kind of dog that's right for your needs, where to acquire it, and how to be sure it is healthy.

Which Breed Is Best?

It is difficult to be definite about which breeds are right in terms of number of children and number of adults, residence in cities or suburbs, apartments, houses, and mobile homes, etc. It is not so much a question of where you live or the amount of space available, but of how much time and effort you are willing to devote to raising, training, feeding, grooming, and most important of all, loving a dog. Dogs can adapt to almost any environment. There are some exceptions, of course. Some breeds may be too difficult to handle or too temperamental for the elderly, the handicapped, or the family with young children. If you live in a one-room apartment and drive a subcompact car, you can anticipate problems owning a St. Bernard, Great Dane, or other giant breed. Choosing a dog involves common sense and preplanning. Don't rush out and impulsively buy or adopt the first cute puppy you see. In *The Good Dog Book,* Mordecai Siegal says that "getting a dog is like having a baby. It is not a simple, casual matter. One must prepare."

The following questions may help you determine what type of dog is right for you:

1. Can you afford to own a dog? Whether you decide on a purebred or mixed-breed dog is a matter of personal preference and aesthetics; the responsibilities and procedures for raising a purebred or mixed breed are the same. Only the purchase price varies. Owning a dog can be expensive. Food and medical care are the major expenditures, but don't forget to consider yearly license fees, toys, collars and leashes, grooming equipment and supplies, boarding fees while you are vacationing, and perhaps obedience training, professional grooming, and show-handling fees.

2. Do you have the time to make the dog a happy addition to the family? No matter what kind of dog you own, it will needs lots of attention. A dog needs to be housebroken and taught to obey basic obedience commands, in addition to getting regular meals, grooming, bathing, exercise, and play periods.

3. What type of dog are you looking for? Will it be a companion, a child's pet, a dog for personal protection or for breeding or showing? Before buying, know positively why you want to own a dog and how the dog will adapt to your life-style.

4. Do you want a small or a large dog? Most dogs can adapt to any environment, but size can be important. Many urban dwellers want dogs for personal protection. If you live in a city apartment and are considering a large or giant breed, think first about how much time you will be able to spend walking and exercising the dog. It is cruel to keep a large animal shut up in a small apartment without adequate exercise.

5. Do you want a smooth- or long-haired dog? Smooth-coated breeds are the easiest to care for and require a

minimum of grooming; long-haired dogs need some kind of regular care. Some long-coated breeds should be brushed daily, while others need to be expertly clipped, scissored, stripped, or plucked regularly. If you do not have the time or the ability to do the necessary trimming, grooming, or bathing at home, it may be expensive to have it done professionally.

6. Do you want a male or female? Males are generally more aggressive, energetic, and more likely to roam, especially when looking for females in season. The female dog's ability to reproduce is determined by her heat cycle, which generally starts when she is 6 to 12 months of age. During each heat cycle or season, which lasts about 21 days the female secretes a blood-tinged discharge which attracts male dogs to mate. Unless puppies are wanted, the female should be isolated from male dogs during heat. Her movements outside should be supervised: she must not be allowed to run free or she may be bred accidentally. Females that have the run of the house may need to wear special sanitary pants during heat to keep discharges from staining furniture or bedding. This may not bother some pet owners, but is felt as an inconvenience by others. These problems can be solved by having the dog spayed or neutered. If you are not buying a dog for breeding, consider having it altered to prevent accidental breeding. Spaying or neutering makes a dog more gentle and affectionate, and is a humane solution for lowering the number of unwanted pets flooding the nation's animal shelters. (For more information on spaying and neutering, see "20 Commonsense Suggestions for Dog Owners.")

For advice on choosing a dog, there are a number of books available that will acquaint you with the purebreds and one charming book devoted to selecting the right mixed-breed dog:

American Kennel Club: *The Complete Dog Book.* Howell Book House, New York, 1979.
Denenberg, R. V., and Seidman, Eric: *The Dog Catalog.* Grosset & Dunlap, New York, 1978.
Dolensek, Nancy, and Burn, Barbara: *Mutt.* Clarkson N. Potter, New York, 1978.
Howe, John: *Choosing the Right Dog: A Buyer's Guide to All 121 Breeds.* Harper & Row, New York, 1976.

Unkelbach, Kurt: *Best of Breeds Guide for Young Dog Lovers.* G. P. Putnam's Sons, New York, 1978.

Go to your library or bookstore and read as much as you can about dogs. If you are interested in a purebred dog, you may have narrowed your choice down to several breeds and need more information to make a final decision. One of the best ways to see breeds is to go to a dog show. (Information about dog shows can be found in your newspaper's calendar of sports events.) Buy a catalog as soon as you arrive at the show: ring locations and scheduled judging times for the various breeds are listed. Also, at a dog show you can meet people who breed and show the dogs in which you are interested. Go to the ringside and watch your favorite breeds being judged. After the judging, introduce yourself to a few exhibitors and indicate that you are interested in owning their breed. Most breeders or exhibitors will acclaim their breed's virtues, but when questioned sincerely, most are willing to give sensible advice to prospective owners. Another way to decide which breed is right for you is to consult a veterinarian, since some purebreds have a tendency to develop certain problems (skin conditions and eye or ear disorders, for example), while others have a high incidence of genetically influenced diseases.

Where to Get a Dog

Most puppies are sold by pet stores. Much has been written about buying a puppy from a pet shop—not all of it complimentary. Pet stores may breed their own puppies, buy puppies from or offer a puppy referral service through local breeders, or buy from kennels or so-called "puppy mills" which mass-produce puppies. It is possible to obtain a good puppy at a pet store, but if the shop buys from kennels which mass-produce and ship off puppies at an early age, the quality of the dogs may be inconsistent. The store owner, who has not seen the sires or dams, may have no idea which puppies have come from healthy, sound, good-tempered parents and have been socialized properly. (See "Puppy Socialization" in section III.)

Dedicated noncommercial breeders are the best source for purebred puppies, especially for breeding or show quality. The serious breeder tries to improve a breed with each generation by breeding puppies that are better than their sires or dams. Quality dogs are seldom produced indiscriminately. It takes hours of planning and research before breeding two animals. The virtues and faults of sire and dam should be evaluated and both pedigrees researched thoroughly. Once breeding takes place, the female must receive the best nutrition and care throughout her pregnancy for the fullest development of her puppies.

Dedicated breeding means having a knowledge of genetics, mating, whelping, weaning, pediatrics, nutrition, health care, early socialization and development of the puppies, evaluating the litter properly, and getting the puppies to the right owners.

The best way to locate breeders is through dog-show catalogs, kennel clubs, and direct contact at dog shows or through advertisements in magazines such as *Pure-Bred Dogs, American Kennel Gazette, Dog World, Kennel Review, Show Dogs, Dogs,* and *Dog Fancy.*

You can get a dog from an animal shelter or adoption agency. Every area has one where you can get a dog for a small fee or voluntary contribution. Dogs (and cats, too) are suffering from overpopulation throughout the world; too many pets are being euthanized at an early age in shelters because there are not enough homes available. Adopting a dog is a humane thing to do, for undoubtedly you will be saving the animal's life.

Many of the dogs in shelters are of mixed ancestry, but a number of purebred dogs are available. If you want to adopt a pet, go to a shelter or adoption agency and take a good look at all the dogs. If you are concerned about a puppy's size, someone there may be able to tell you how big the dog will get to be. Spend time choosing the right puppy, and don't forget that a shelter atmosphere affects dogs, making some shy or intimidated and others noisy or assertive (often out of fright). You may be in for some surprises after you bring the puppy home, but remember that almost every dog will be happier, more adaptable, and more sociable after several weeks in a new home.

Selecting a Healthy Puppy

Don't buy on impulse. Every puppy is cute and cuddly, but consider that you are about to embark on a 10-to-15-year period of togetherness with a dog. A little planning and investigation can help you select a healthy, good-tempered animal.

Age is important. The best time to buy a pet is when a puppy is 6 to 8 weeks old—the best time for a puppy to adapt to its new owner and environment. On the other hand, this is too young to buy a puppy for show or breeding purposes. The older a puppy is the more you can tell about its conformation, which is important when purchasing a future stud dog, brood matron, or show dog.

Ask to see the whole litter at one time. Watch the puppies romp and play together. If one seems appealing, watch it closely. How does the puppy behave with its littermates? Is it bold and friendly? Is it curious? Is it overly shy, frightened, or nervous? Does it come up to you? Does it run away when you make a noise? *Temperament is of the utmost importance.* Nervous or shy puppies may experience behavior problems as adults. The puppy that is friendly, outgoing, and interested in its littermates and in you is the one you should choose.

Ask to see the mother of the puppies (and the father as well, if he is available). There is a saying that "if you want to see how a girl will mature, take a look at her mother." With modifications, this can be applied to pure-bred dogs. You can tell a great deal about the way a puppy will mature by seeing its dam and sire. If the parents are friendly and even-tempered, odds are that the puppies will be too. If they are nervous, shy, or overly aggressive, consider looking elsewhere for a puppy.

Signs of healthy puppies include the following:

1. The eyes should be clear and bright, with no discharge or sensitivity to light.
2. The ears should be clean and pleasant-smelling. There should be no indications of scratching or head shaking. To test for deafness, clap your hands behind the puppy and see if it responds.
3. The nose should be moist, with no discharge.
4. The baby teeth should be white, not pitted or stained. The gums should be pink and firm. Pale pink or

whitish gums indicate anemia, which may be caused by a heavy worm infestation. The puppy's breath should smell pleasant.

5. The coat should be glossy with no bare spots. There should be no indication of skin disease or external parasites.

6. The puppy should be in good flesh—not too fat or too thin, with ribs exposed. Avoid puppies with distended bellies, which can mean internal parasites.

7. The puppy should be lively, active, and interested in its littermates and surroundings.

Signs of a sick puppy include:

1. Dull, dry coat
2. Distended or "pot" belly
3. Diarrhea or bloody stools
4. Discharge from eyes or nose
5. Eyes sensitive to light
6. Coughing
7. Excessive head shaking or scratching the ears
8. Pale pink or whitish gums
9. Sluggish or lethargic behavior

Don't be afraid to ask for a health guarantee. A reliable breeder or pet store will not hesitate to offer a written guarantee that the puppy can be returned within a specific time limit if it shows any symptoms of illness. Once the puppy is purchased, it is the new owner's responsibility to have the puppy examined by a veterinarian as soon as possible.

Don't hesitate to ask pertinent questions or do not be upset when the breeder questions you. As you are searching for the right puppy, the breeder is looking closely at you to determine how the puppy will fit into your lifestyle and if you are buying on impulse or are really serious about giving the puppy the love, attention, and care it requires.

Once you buy a puppy, the breeder or pet store should provide the following:

1. A record of the puppy's temporary and/or permanent immunization against distemper, hepatitis, leptospirosis, etc., and the dates when future inoculations or boosters are due

2. A health record, including the dates of wormings
3. Information about feeding the puppy

If the puppy is a purebred, you should receive the American Kennel Club registration paper and a three-to-five-generation pedigree. An inexperienced puppy buyer may misinterpret the words "pedigree" and "papers." A pedigree lists the father, mother, grandparents, great-grandparents, and other ancestors from which a dog descends. It is a dog's genealogical record. The registration paper is an application for registration issued by the AKC. It indicates that your dog was a product of a registered purebred sire and a dam of the same breed in a litter that was registered. When you buy a puppy eligible for AKC registration, you are entitled to receive an AKC application from the seller which will allow you to register the dog in your name. The rules and regulations of the AKC specify that when someone sells a dog eligible for AKC registration, the seller must identify the dog either by giving the buyer a properly completed AKC registration paper, or if the paper is not yet available, a bill of sale or written statement signed by the seller and giving the following information:

a. The puppy's breed, sex, and color.
b. The puppy's date of birth.
c. The registered names of the puppy's sire and dam.
d. The breeder's name.

Remember: When you buy a purebred puppy, you should get either the AKC registration paper or a bill of sale with a written statement containing the above information. *Don't accept a promise of later identification.* For more information about buying a dog and AKC registration, you may wish to write to the American Kennel Club, 51 Madison Avenue, New York, NY 10010, and request a copy of their pamphlet, *Are You a Responsible Dog Owner?*

Buying a puppy is a memorable experience. Careful selection of the right puppy is important, since you and your family are making a commitment to living with a dog for a number of years. With a little planning and searching, it's possible to locate the right puppy and have it become a highly regarded, well-adjusted member of your family.

YOUR DOG'S HEALTH

From the day you whelp or buy a puppy, its physical health depends on two people—you and your veterinarian—and an exchange of information that will be important to the dog's welfare.

Selecting a Veterinarian

The best way to ensure your dog's good health is to select a veterinarian in whom you have confidence, as carefully and deliberately as you choose a family doctor. If you need help, ask for recommendations from dog breeders or exhibitors and pet stores in your area or the local veterinary association.

Once you have made a tentative selection, make a visit to his or her veterinary hospital and check out the following questions:

1. Is the hospital conveniently located? (An important consideration in an emergency, for instance, is to be able to reach a veterinarian quickly.)

2. Are the reception area and treatment rooms scrupulously clean? A veterinary hospital or office should have a positive environment. As soon as you enter, the atmosphere of the reception area should convey the impression that the hospital is reliable and that the employees are trustworthy. A dirty reception area or one filled with offensive smells does not instill confidence. When you go into the treatment room, has the examining table been disinfected after the previous animal? Does the room project a sterile "hospital" atmosphere?

3. Are the staff kind and considerate to animals? Do they appear to be knowledgeable or uninterested? Every employee should give you the feeling that if your dog had to stay overnight, it would receive reliable care.

4. What are the regular office hours and the veterinarian's day off? How does he or she manage emergencies? It's important to know how fast medical attention is available after an emergency. This does not mean that you should be able to bother your veterinarian at home with trivial problems that can be treated during regular office hours, but it does mean that you can reach him or her

(and not a telephone recording) in a life-threatening emergency. *Accidents and emergencies can occur at any hour of the day. No seriously injured dog should have to suffer needlessly or die because it's the veterinarian's day off or after regular hours.*

5. Does the veterinarian handle your dog gently and firmly? How does the dog respond to the handling? You are seeking someone who is competent, but it's nice to have a veterinarian who loves animals too.

6. Is it possible to exchange thoughts or suggestions about the dog's welfare or does the veterinarian have an uninterested manner? Do you feel that a good working relationship can be developed?

Remember, the relationship is not one-sided. Your veterinarian has the right to expect certain things from you, such as being considerate and knowledgeable. Most veterinarians have large practices and are too busy to be disturbed during office hours with unimportant questions or after regular hours with minor problems. Learn to be considerate about using your veterinarian's services, but don't hesitate to call when it's really necessary. Get to know your dog as an individual. Once you understand what is normal for your dog, you will learn to recognize changes in behavior or general condition that indicate potential trouble. Learn to observe your dog's symptoms and to describe them accurately to your veterinarian.

If you expect competent treatment, be prepared to pay accordingly. Veterinarians receive a great deal of specialized training and the hospital equipment, surgical procedures, and medicines used are similar to those used on humans.

Every 6 to 7 months, take your dog for a general checkup. More and more veterinarians recommend semiannual examinations, on the theory that early detection and treatment can prolong life. Dogs should have more frequent health examinations than people, since they mature almost five times as fast. At a regular examination take along a fresh stool sample and have the veterinarian make a laboratory fecal examination for worms. Internal parasites are a common problem among dogs; when they are neglected, serious problems, especially anemia, can result. Dogs should have annual booster shots for certain infectious diseases.

It is your responsibility as well as the veterinarian's to keep your dog as healthy as possible. You should know about vaccinations, internal parasites, external parasites, skin problems, grooming, and other phases of health care.

IMMUNIZATION AGAINST INFECTIOUS DISEASES

During the first 24 hours of its life, a nursing puppy receives protective antibodies from its mother's milk, or colostrum, which protect it against certain diseases (to which the mother is immune) for several weeks. Temporary protection can last 2 to 12 weeks and even longer, depending on the mother's immunity. Most veterinarians begin vaccination at 8 weeks of age, giving a puppy two or three injections between 8 and 16 weeks of age. Until the immunization program is complete, keep puppies isolated from other dogs or sources of infectious disease. The veterinarian can take a blood serum test from the mother to determine the exact level of the puppy's maternal immunity and predict the best time to immunize, but this is expensive. Dogs should be immunized against canine distemper, infectious canine hepatitis, leptospirosis, infectious tracheobronchitis, canine parvovirus, and rabies.

Canine Distemper

Distemper is a common disease which destroys many dogs each year. Young dogs are the most susceptible, but older dogs can be infected. Distemper, a virus disease, is spread by air, contact with an infected animal, or contaminated objects such as clothing, bedding, food pans, cages, and carrying cases. Canine distemper is not transmissible to man. The incubation period, from exposure to the virus to development of symptoms, is 4 to 9 days. Symptoms include:

1. Elevated temperature, often as high as 105°F (40.5°C)
2. Watery discharge from the eyes and nose which gradually thickens and changes to pus
3. The eyes blink a great deal and become sensitive to light

4. Crusts form around the nostrils
5. Pads of the feet may thicken and harden
6. Poor appetite
7. Listlessness
8. Chronic vomiting and diarrhea, which can cause rapid dehydration and weight loss
9. Coughing
10. The dog may develop pneumonia as a result of a secondary bacterial infection
11. Muscle twitching
12. Convulsions

Any or all of these symptoms may appear; in the early phases it may be difficult to distinguish distemper from other diseases.

Distemper has a high mortality rate, but many dogs recover to live a normal, happy life. Survivors are sometimes left with pitted, discolored teeth and nervous aftereffects, such as muscle twitching of various parts of the body (*chorea*).

A dog suspected of having distemper should receive veterinary attention immediately. The sooner treatment is begun, the greater the chance of recovery, although there is no treatment effective against the distemper virus. Therapy consists of limiting secondary bacterial infections and supporting the general health of the patient. Antibiotics, anticonvulsants, antidiarrhea medications, and dietary supplements may be prescribed. You will probably be responsible for most of your dog's therapy at home, since many veterinarians do not want to hospitalize distempered dogs for fear of infecting other animals. Good home nursing care, love, and a positive attitude can be a great help to the recovering dog. (See section II, "Home Nursing," for additional suggestions to help make your dog more comfortable during convalescence.) Animals that have recovered from distemper are thought to be immune, but a yearly booster should be given to be absolutely sure.

Immunization (usually combined with immunization against other canine diseases) is the best way to prevent distemper. Several types of vaccines are used; selection of vaccine and inoculation schedule will depend on your veterinarian and his or her experience in controlling the disease in your area.

Infectious Canine Hepatitis

Infectious canine hepatitis destroys many dogs each year. Again, young animals are more susceptible. The disease is caused by a virus and is spread by contact with the urine, feces, or saliva of an infected animal. The virus is different from the one that causes hepatitis in humans and the canine disease does not affect humans. The incubation period is 6 to 9 days. Symptoms of infectious canine hepatitis include:

1. Elevated temperature—often as high as 105°F to 106°F (40.5°C to 41°C). Temperature often rises for a day, then falls back to almost normal for a day, then rises again
2. Loss of appetite
3. Excessive thirst
4. Watery discharge from the eyes and nose which gradually thickens and changes to pus
5. Bloody diarrhea
6. Blood in vomit
7. Tender and painful abdomen. The abdomen may be so painful from enlargement of the liver that the dog's body appears to be drawn together and humpbacked
8. Mucous membranes of the mouth may be red
9. Tonsils may be enlarged
10. There may be a blue cloudiness in one or both eyes. "Blue eye" is associated with or follows some forms of canine hepatitis. It is not painful and generally, but not always, disappears naturally. Blue eye occurs (much less frequently) in dogs that have been vaccinated against canine hepatitis

It is difficult to distinguish between early hepatitis and distemper. Hepatitis is often fatal, but many dogs recover to live normal lives. A recovered animal eliminates hepatitis virus in its urine for some time, which is one way the disease is spread.

If you suspect your dog has hepatitis, it should receive veterinary attention immediately. The sooner treatment is begun, the greater the chance of recovery. Dogs with hepatitis usually have to be hospitalized. Controlling hemorrhage is often a problem (there is a direct relationship between the seriousness of hepatitis and clotting time), and blood transfusions may be necessary.

When the dog comes home from the hospital, competent nursing care and a positive attitude can play an important part toward recovery. (See section II, "Home Nursing," for suggestions to help make your dog more comfortable during convalescence.)

Immunization, usually combined with immunization against other canine diseases, is the best way to prevent infectious canine hepatitis.

Leptospirosis

Leptospirosis is a spirochete infection caused by two species of bacteria, *Leptospira canicola* and *Leptospira icterohaemorrhagiae*, that attack the kidneys and liver. The disease occurs in dogs, horses, cattle and other farm animals, rats and other rodents, and some wild animals. It is transmissible to man (in whom the diseases are known as canicola fever and Weil's disease, respectively). Both diseases are spread through the urine of infected animals. Spirochetes enter the body following contamination of the mucous membranes of the mouth or nose with infected urine, or less often through openings in the skin or during breeding. *Leptospira icterohaemorrhagiae* is transmitted through rat urine; if the disease appears in your dog, rat infestation in home or kennel should be controlled immediately, especially in food storage areas.

The incubation period is 5 to 15 days. Symptoms of leptospirosis include:

1. Sudden elevated temperature, as high as 105°F (40.5°C), at the onset. Within 2 days there is a sudden drop in temperature
2. Loss of appetite
3. Labored breathing
4. Depression
5. Urine may be dark yellow or orange in color and have a strong smell
6. Mucous membranes of the mouth may have patches resembling burns or abrasions which later dry and peel off in sections
7. Tenderness and pain in the abdominal area
8. Stiffness and soreness of the hind legs, especially when attempting to rise from a sitting position

9. If the disease was acquired from a rat, there may be symptoms of jaundice

In advanced cases:

1. The dog is very depressed
2. Temperature can drop gradually to as low as 97°F (36°C)
3. There is bloody vomiting and diarrhea, which can cause rapid dehydration and weight loss
4. The dog is unusually thirsty and urinates frequently
5. The eyes may become sunken
6. There may be muscle twitching

Dogs of all ages are susceptible to leptospirosis, which occurs more frequently in males. It can be fatal, but many dogs recover to lead normal lives. It may be difficult to diagnose leptospirosis in the early stages.

If you suspect your dog has leptospirosis, contact your veterinarian immediately, for if treatment is begun before the spirochetes permanently damage the kidneys and liver, the chances of recovery are greater. Hospitalization is necessary and treatment consists of antibiotics, fluid therapy, dietary supplements, and sometimes blood transfusions. When the dog comes home from the hospital, competent nursing care, lots of love, and a positive attitude will play an important part in recovery. After the dog has recovered from leptospirosis, the spirochetes can be eliminated in its urine for months.

Immunization is the best way to prevent leptospirosis. The immunizing agent is not a vaccine but a bacterin, usually combined with immunization against other canine diseases. Duration of immunity is shorter, however, and in areas where exposure risk is above average, immunization against leptospirosis may be necessary every 6 months instead of once a year. Consult your veterinarian.

Infectious Tracheobronchitis

Tracheobronchitis is an infectious respiratory disease in dogs caused by a parainfluenza virus. The disease is often called "kennel cough," because dogs that are kept in kennels, hospitals, pet shops, or animal shelters are often infected by diseased animals or contaminated areas or articles. The virus spreads rapidly from dog to dog; dogs of any age are susceptible.

Symptoms include a dry, hacking cough which may be followed by heaving motions accompanied by a white, foamy secretion from the mouth. Partial obstruction of the airway causes the dog to act like something is stuck in its throat. External palpation of the larynx or trachea intensifies the coughing. The dog may vomit occasionally.

Infectious tracheobronchitis should be treated promptly, for if the condition is neglected, serious complications such as pneumonia can develop. Do not attempt home treatment. A cough can be a symptom of many diseases other than tracheobronchitis, and it is important that the dog be diagnosed and treated by a veterinarian.

Dogs with mild cases recover in 1 to 3 weeks, with longer recovery for dogs that develop a secondary infection such as pneumonia. Treatment includes use of antibiotics to treat secondary infection, cough suppressants to control coughing, and bronchodilators to help reduce swelling and irritation. The dog can recuperate at home in a warm, dry atmosphere, but it must be isolated from other family pets to prevent the disease from spreading. Good nursing care, careful sanitary procedures, and good nutrition will help encourage your dog's recovery.

Modified live canine parainfluenza virus vaccine is available to control the causative agents in infectious tracheobronchitis. Vaccination is recommended by 8 weeks of age. The parainfluenza vaccine is usually combined with distemper hepatitis vaccines and leptospirosis bacterin and given in the same injection. Other viruses that cause respiratory disease in dogs are not included in the immunity provided by canine parainfluenza vaccine. Annual booster shots are recommended: these are especially important if your dog is to be boarded in a kennel while you are away from home.

Canine Parvovirus

Canine parvovirus (CPV) is a new disease-producing agent of dogs, first identified in the United States in 1978, that occurs throughout the world. Two CPV forms are seen: enteritis in dogs of all ages and the rarer myocarditis in young puppies. The enteric form attacks dogs suddenly between 3 to 12 days after exposure, and symptoms begin with depression and loss of appetite. These are swiftly followed by vomiting and gray (often bloody) diarrhea. The temperature may go beyond 104°F and death can occur within 24 hours after the onset of symptoms. This extremely contagious virus is spread primarily through the feces of infected animals. The myocardial form is usually seen in puppies of less than 3 months of age. The virus attacks the muscle cells of the heart. Affected puppies are often found dead or die within hours after experiencing periods of difficult breathing. Those that survive may endure permanent heart damage.

Dogs infected with parvovirus need immediate veterinary care. Treatment for the enteric form involves control of the vomiting and diarrhea and the injection of intravenous or subcutaneous fluids to counteract dehydration. Most dogs recover within a week to ten days if they receive early treatment. Infected dogs should be isolated. CPV is not only extremely contagious but also hard to destroy. It can withstand freezing and thawing, temperatures over 120°F (for several days), alcohol, and most disinfectants. The only agents known to destroy canine parvovirus are chlorox (1:30 dilution) and formaldehyde.

Immunization is the recommended method of controlling CPV. Soon after the disease was recognized, its similarity to feline panleukopenia virus (FPV), or cat distemper, was noted. Researchers of the Baker Institute for Animal Health at Cornell University discovered that FPV vaccines would protect dogs against canine parvovirus. New vaccines were eventually developed for commercial use in dogs. The vaccine should be part of your immunization program. Yearly boosters are recommended.

Rabies

Rabies is a viral infection that occurs in dogs, cats, bats, skunks, foxes, raccoons, wolves, and coyotes. All warm-blooded animals are susceptible to rabies and the disease is transmissible to man. The virus is found in an infected animal's saliva and is spread by its bite, or if saliva contacts any break in the skin by other means.

The incubation period is 10 to 50 days or longer in

SUGGESTED VACCINATIONS

Disease	Type of Vaccine Used[a]	When to Vaccinate[b]
Canine distemper	Modified live canine distemper virus vaccine, or modified live measles/virus vaccine	*Puppies:* First vaccination at about 8 weeks of age. Second vaccination at 12–16 weeks of age. If the mother is not immune to distemper, the puppies will receive no protective antibodies from her and should receive globulin or measles vaccine as soon as possible. Measles vaccine can be given as early as 6 weeks of age. At 12–16 weeks of age, vaccinate with canine distemper virus vaccine. *Adults:* Revaccinate annually.
Infectious canine hepatitis	Modified live infectious canine hepatitis virus vaccine, or inactivated vaccine	*Puppies:* First vaccination at about 8 weeks of age. Second vaccination at 12–16 weeks of age. Usually combined with canine distemper virus vaccine and given in one injection. *Adults:* Revaccinate annually.
Canine leptospirosis (two types: *Leptospira canicola* and *L. icterohaemmorrhagiae*)	Killed bacteria (not a vaccine but a bacterin)	*Puppies:* First vaccination at about 8 weeks of age. Second vaccination at 12–16 weeks of age. Vaccines for both types can be given separately or combined with distemper and hepatitis vaccines and given in one injection. *Adults:* Revaccinate annually. In areas where leptospirosis risk is greater than normal, inoculations every 6 months may be advised; consult your veterinarian.

Infectious tracheo-bronchitis	Modified live canine parainfluenza vaccine	*Puppies:* Usually combined with distemper and hepatitis vaccines and leptospirosis bacterin and given in one injection.
		Adults: Revaccinate annually.
Canine parvovirus	Modified live virus vaccine	*Puppies:* First vaccination at about 8 weeks of age. Second vaccination at about 10 to 12 weeks of age. Third booster two weeks later.
		Adults: Revaccinate annually.
Rabies	Modified live rabies virus	*Puppies:* First vaccination is given when puppy is 3–4 months old.
		Adults: Revaccinate at 1 year of age, then once every three years—even if puppy is over 4 months of age at first vaccination.
	Inactivated virus	*Puppies:* First vaccination is given when the puppy is 3–4 months old. Second vaccination is given 3–4 weeks later.
		Adults: Revaccinate annually.

[a] Several types of vaccines are used for immunization. Selection of type of vaccine and your dog's inoculation schedule will depend on your veterinarian and his or her experience in controlling these diseases in your area. Vaccination programs may vary among veterinarians, but the principles remain the same.

[b] A puppy usually will get several vaccinations before immunity is complete. A great many pet owners are not aware that even after a puppy is immunized, annual revaccination is necessary.

some cases, depending on several factors, including the location and severity of the bite. The virus is carried to the central nervous system and eventually travels to the brain and salivary glands. The closer the bite is to the brain, the sooner the symptoms manifest themselves. A bite on the face or head may produce symptoms in the minimum 10 days.

There are two forms of the disease, "furious rabies" and "dumb or paralytic rabies"; the second form can be distinct or can follow the furious form. The most common symptom of the disease in its early stages is a change in the dog's behavior: it may stop eating and drinking and be withdrawn, looking for seclusion. After 1 to 3 days, infected animals either become aggressive and vicious or exhibit symptoms of paralysis.

The furious form of rabies causes the infected animal to become vicious and disposed to attack. Symptoms include:

1. No paralysis in the early stages
2. Dilated eye pupils
3. Noises or bright lights can bring about an attack. An infected animal is eager to bite. Dogs with furious rabies often wander the streets and violently attack people, other animals, or moving objects

As the disease progresses:

4. There is a progressive loss of muscular control
5. Convulsions become common. The dog may die during a seizure or progress into the dumb or paralytic form

After the onset of symptoms, infected dogs seldom live longer than 10 days.

Symptoms of dumb or paralytic rabies include:

1. Early paralysis of the mouth and throat muscles
2. Inability to swallow. The dog cannot eat or drink and becomes dehydrated
3. The lower jaw drops open
4. There is excess salivation, caused by the difficulty in swallowing; it is not "hydrophobia" or frothing at the mouth

Dogs with this form of rabies generally are not ferocious and do not try to bite. The paralysis spreads quickly to other areas of the body and the dog becomes comatose and dies within a few hours.

If your dog is bitten by an animal *suspected* of suffering from rabies, that animal should be captured and confined —but remember to protect yourself from being bitten. If necessary, call your local ASPCA or Humane Society for help in capturing the rabies suspect. Notify your Public Health officials as they will want to quarantine the suspect for observation. If no symptoms develop, the animal will be released.

If your dog has an up-to-date rabies vaccination and is bitten by a *known* rabid animal, have it revaccinated and keep it under close observation for about 3 months. An unvaccinated dog bitten by an animal *known* to have rabies may have to be euthanized, or if you do not want the dog put to sleep, it should be vaccinated and isolated for 6 months.

A current rabies vaccination is the only way to confer immunity. Since rabies is transmissible to and dangerous to man, dogs are subject to state and local ordinances on rabies control. In many areas you must present a current rabies vaccination certificate to obtain a dog license. Selection of type of vaccine and inoculation schedule against rabies depends on your veterinarian and local or state regulations.

The chart is a guide to suggested vaccinations (pp. 292–293).

INTERNAL PARASITES

Internal parasites are a common problem among dogs; if neglected, serious problems can result because the dog's physical condition will deteriorate rapidly. The most common external parasites are roundworms, hookworms, whipworms, tapeworms, and heartworms. Coccidiosis, an intestinal infection caused by a minute protozoan organism, is also common in dogs.

Roundworms

The two species of roundworms that infest dogs are *Toxocara canis* and *Toxascaris leonina,* the former mostly in puppies and young dogs and the latter mostly in mature dogs. The species can be distinguished by identifying their eggs. Adult roundworms are white, 1/16th inch in diameter, and 2 to 6 inches long.

The life cycle of the roundworm is complex. Dogs can become infested after ingesting roundworm eggs from contaminated soil. Following ingestion, the eggs hatch in the upper small intestine, penetrate the intestinal wall, and enter the bloodstream where they reach the right chambers of the heart. Then they migrate to the pulmonary arteries and into the lungs. They continue to grow as they ascend the respiratory tract and are coughed up and reswallowed, returning to the small intestine to complete their maturity. Once mature, adult females can lay several thousand eggs per day which pass in the dog's stool.

Some of the roundworm larvae in the lungs are not coughed up and reswallowed but return to the right chamber of the heart to be distributed to various body organs and tissues where they become encapsulated and lie dormant. During pregnancy, some of the dormant larvae become active and may cross the placenta and enter the fetus. After birth, the larvae migrate to the new puppy's intestines and mature. Larvae can also be transmitted to nursing puppies via their mother's milk. If puppies are infested before birth or while nursing, they can pass roundworm eggs at 3 weeks of age. Puppies also can become infested with roundworms by eating stool or dirt contaminated with eggs.

Roundworm infestation is especially debilitating to puppies. Symptoms include overall weakness, malnutrition, and dull hair coat. The puppy may be ravenous but remain thin and develop a potbellied or distended abdomen. Infested puppies have respiratory difficulties and discharges from the eyes. They may cough and often vomit a few roundworms, or have diarrhea and pass roundworms in the stool.

Diagnosis of roundworms should be made by your veterinarian. A number of products are safe and effective against roundworm, for example, Piperazine and Pyrantel

Pamoate, which require no fasting before administration. Worming should be done by your veterinarian or under his or her supervision. Usually a second (and possibly a third) worming will be necessary in 2 to 4 weeks.

Roundworms have public health significance, since the larvae can cause visceral larva migrans in humans, especially children. Infestation is as in the dog, by ingestion of eggs which hatch in the intestines, penetrate the intestinal wall, and reach the bloodstream. Larvae do not go to the human lungs, however, but migrate throughout the body, causing considerable damage which can be debilitating. If the larvae migrate into the eye, they can cause permanent damage. Infestation often results when children and infested dogs live and play in the same areas. Ingestion can occur when a child eats egg-infested soil or touches contaminated dirt or infested dog feces and then puts the hands in the mouth.

Hookworms

Hookworms are small parasites which become attached to the dog's intestinal wall and suck its blood. Adult hookworms are grayish and $1/4$ to $1/2$ inch long. Infestation occurs through mouth or skin penetration. If the larvae enter by mouth, they penetrate the wall of the small intestine and migrate through the bloodstream to the lungs. In a few days, they are coughed up, reswallowed, and reach the small intestine a second time where they mature into adult worms. If the larvae enter by penetrating the skin, they also migrate through the bloodstream to the lungs, are coughed up, swallowed, and reach the small intestine where they mature into adult worms. The maturation process takes 18 to 21 days; then adult females living in the intestines can lay several thousand eggs a day. The eggs are passed in the dog's feces, and under optimum conditions can hatch in 48 to 72 hours, releasing larvae which develop into the infestive stage in 5 to 7 days.

Some larvae penetrating the skin may reach the circulatory system and be carried to various body organs where they lie dormant. During pregnancy the larvae can become active, cross the placenta, and infest the developing fetus. Larvae also can be transmitted to nursing puppies via their mother's milk.

Symptoms of hookworm infestation can vary from absence of vigorous growth (unthriftiness) to fatal anemia, depending on the severity of the infestation and the dog's age and physical condition. The primary sign is anemia. Infested dogs are weak, thin, unthrifty-looking, have dull coats and pale mucous membranes. In young puppies exposed to a heavy infestation of larvae, the first noticeable sign may be pneumonia, immediately followed by anemia and black stools, a result of blood in the intestinal tract.

Diagnosis of hookworm should be made by your veterinarian. The dog should be wormed and fed a well-balanced diet while being maintained in sanitary surroundings.

Whipworms

Whipworms are common in dogs 6 to 24 months old but can be seen in dogs of any age. They are found in the colon and the cecum (the cul-de-sac where the large intestine begins), where the whipworm's head becomes embedded in the intestinal wall. The worms are creamy-colored, grow to about 2 inches long, and are shaped like a whip. They complete their life cycle in the intestinal area and pass eggs in the dog's feces.

A light infestation of whipworm produces no specific signs, but as the infestation increases diarrhea and loss of weight may be noticed. The stools of heavily infested dogs may contain fresh blood. Diagnosis and treatment of whipworm should be done by your veterinarian. Whipworm eggs require a warm moist environment to develop; therefore, keeping your dog's living quarters or kennel clean, dry, and reasonably cool will help reduce infestation.

Tapeworms

Several forms of tapeworm are seen in the dog, the most common of which include:

1. *Dipylidium caninum,* acquired from fleas or, rarely, lice—the most common dog tapeworm. The flea or the louse consumes the tapeworm larva, which can be ingested by a dog that is infested with fleas (or lice) and bites its skin for relief. Once ingested, the tapeworm

larvae migrate to the dog's intestines where they attach themselves to the intestinal wall and grow a series of flat connected segments.

2. *Taenia pisiformis,* acquired by eating raw meat or the internal tissues and organs of rabbits, sheep, goats, pigs, squirrels, and some rodents. This type is more common among suburban, farm, and hunting dogs.

3. *Diphyllobothrium* species, acquired by eating the body and organs of certain raw infected fish. This type is found in Canada, Alaska, and some parts of the United States.

Tapeworms are common in dogs, especially strays and dogs that are permitted to run free. About 20% of the stray dogs (and cats) in this country are infested.

Adult tapeworms are creamy and can grow to a length of several feet. The tapeworm's head attaches itself to the intestinal wall, making it hard to dislodge: the neck frequently breaks off, leaving the head intact to regenerate a new body. Segments of a mature tapeworm containing eggs often break off and pass out in the dog's feces. They can be seen moving in the stool, or they can dry in the hair or on the skin around the anus and look like rice kernels.

Symptoms of tapeworm are not well defined and vary with species type, severity of infestation, and age and physical condition of the dog; however, they can include unthriftiness, poor hair coat, erratic appetite, weakness and listlessness, a mild form of diarrhea, and sometimes abnormal thinness.

Treatment for tapeworm should be prescribed by a veterinarian. To cure tapeworm you must not only rid the dog of the worms, but control the intermediate host, especially the flea, to prevent reinfestation.

Guidelines for Worming

When internal parasites are suspected, your veterinarian can determine the type of worm through microscopic study of a fresh sample of the dog's feces. (See "Collecting Fecal and Urine Samples" in section II.) The stool sample must be fresh for accurate identification of eggs. Once the worm has been identified, your veterinarian can begin correct treatment:

1. Treat the infestation with a safe, effective drug. Be sure your veterinarian has identified the type of parasite before a worming preparation is administered. Many animals are killed every year by indiscriminate worming. Administer over-the-counter preparations only when you know the type of worm present; some wormers can be toxic when used incorrectly or too often.

2. Do not worm a dog with an elevated temperature.

3. Do not worm a sick or debilitated dog.

4. Do not worm a dog that is constipated. Give a mild laxative, such as Milk of Magnesia, a day or 2 before worming.

5. Follow your veterinarian's instructions exactly when giving worm medications. Certain worm medications require fasting before or after dosing; it is important that you follow directions carefully for best results.

6. The most important task is to prevent reinfestation. Generally the dog's environment is the primary source of reinfestation; therefore, it is necessary to keep living quarters or kennel runs scrupulously clean. Remove droppings of stool immediately. Wash the dog's bedding and scald food and water pans. Keep a close check on the dog and its environment for signs of fleas (the intermediate host of tapeworm) and learn how to control these external parasites in your home and yard to prevent reinfestation.

A new drug that treats roundworm and hookworm in dogs, Pyrantel Pamoate, has recently been approved by the Food and Drug Administration for over-the-counter sale. It has been used successfully on large animals and is now approved for canine use. It is available in Lambert Kay's Evict™ Liquid Wormer, an oral suspension that can be given the dog as a treat or added to its food. When used as directed, Pyrantel Pamoate is nontoxic and highly effective. It can be administered to dogs on heartworm medication, dogs recently vaccinated, dogs wearing flea and tick collars, or dogs exposed to organophosphate flea and tick dips. More importantly, it can be used on pregnant bitches and nursing or weaned puppies as well as adult dogs. It does not require fasting before or after dosing and does not produce troublesome side effects such as vomiting or diarrhea.

However, we do not advise the use of an over-the-counter worming remedy without consulting your veterinarian.

Canine Heartworms

Heartworm, which used to be confined to the southern United States, has become widespread. It is passed from dog to dog by mosquitoes, which means that areas with mosquito problems are likely to have a high heartworm rate. When a mosquito bites an infested dog, it takes up blood containing microfilariae (a larval stage of heartworm). When the infested mosquito bites another dog, the larvae are deposited in the dog's bloodstream and migrate to the heart. They lodge in the right chamber of the heart, the venae cavae, and the pulmonary artery and grow to adult size (6 to 14 inches long). Within 5 to 6 months they reach full maturity as reproductive heartworms. Eggs are fertilized and develop in the adult female. Each female can produce up to 30,000 microfilariae per day; these are discharged into the bloodstream where they may be active for a year or more. The microfiliariae in the bloodstream can then be picked up when a mosquito bites the dog.

Heartworms obstruct the flow of blood to the heart and can affect the lungs, kidneys, and liver. Symptoms include fatigue, chronic cough, dull hair coat, eye or nose discharge, and shortness of breath. Fatigue is one of the first noticeable signs, especially in active animals. As the disease progresses, coughing is aggravated by exercise.

Diagnosis involves taking blood samples and X rays. If the test is positive, there are effective drugs which will kill heartworms; when diagnosed early, a dog can be treated successfully. If your dog does not have heartworm or has been returned to the negative state, a drug is available that will prevent microfiliariae from developing into adult heartworms. It is available only from licensed veterinarians and is administered daily in pill form or in the dog's food.

If you live in a heavily infested mosquito area, check with your veterinarian about making the heartworm blood test part of your dog's regular checkup.

Coccidiosis

Coccidiosis is a highly infectious disease caused by a minute protozoan organism living in the lining of the small intestines. It occurs most often in puppies, and is characterized by mild to severe loose stool which is vile-smelling and often contains blood. If the condition is ignored, loss of appetite, depression, and fever will follow. Young dogs infected with coccidia quickly become weak and emaciated.

Coccidia complete their life cycle in the intestines and their eggs are discharged in an infested dog's feces. Once outside the host, the eggs can be picked up easily when another dog walks through a contaminated area and licks its foot pads. Flies can carry coccidia to food pans. When sanitation is poor, puppies can be infested by contact with their mother's stools, or an animal can become reinfested by contact with its own stool.

Your veterinarian may prescribe sulfa drugs or antibiotics to treat coccidiosis; strict sanitation at home is also essential to control the disease and prevent reinfestation. The dog's food pans, living quarters, or kennel runs should be kept clean and disinfected. All stools from infested dogs should be picked up and removed immediately.

EXTERNAL PARASITES

Fleas and ticks, the most common external parasites, can infest dogs at any time of the year. They are a serious direct health problem to your pet, and when a dog is neglected and allowed to become heavily infested, it is susceptible to other serious illnesses because of its debilitated condition. Fleas and ticks live on a dog just long enough to bite it and acquire the necessary blood for reproduction. Adult female fleas lay eggs loose on the dog's body; they fall off on the floor or in the dog's bedding to hatch. Female ticks drop off the dog after breeding and look for quiet places in the house (or kennel) to deposit their eggs: in carpeting and drapes, under the furniture, in the dog's bedding, and in the baseboards or floor cracks and crevices. The hatched flea and tick eggs mature and wait for a host to infest or reinfest. Eventually your house, yard, or kennel can become an incubator for eggs and larvae.

Understanding the life cycles of fleas and ticks is important for their control. There are products that will effectively control fleas and ticks on the dog, but this is only part of the program. The other and more important part is control of larvae in your home, yard, or kennel.

Fleas

Fleas are small brown bloodsucking parasites. They can be detected easily on smooth-coated dogs, but are often hard to see on long-coated pets. The first sign may be a quick glimpse of a dark bug scurrying through the coat or the presence of small black specks on the skin or in the hair. The specks are flea excrement, the end product mostly of blood sucked from the dog. Fleas don't stay in one place for long and their amazing jumping talents make control difficult.

The flea's life cycle has four stages: egg, larva, pupa, and adult. The eggs hatch into larvae in 2 to 12 days, depending on the temperature and humidity. The larvae grow in dark warm places (carpeting, etc.), feeding on food crumbs and animal hairs. When they are developed, the larvae spin small cocoons, and within a few days to several weeks (depending on the weather) hatch into hungry adult fleas.

Flea bites can be serious. The flea bites by sticking its syringelike mouth into the dog's skin and pumping the blood into its stomach. During feeding, the flea secretes saliva into the dog's skin, which causes severe itching. Dogs often develop hypersensitivity to flea saliva which can result in a chronic condition, flea allergy dermatitis, in which the dog's fierce scratching and biting produces loss of hair and causes the skin to become thick, red, and infected. This tends to occur most often on the back, just in front of the tail, on the abdomen, and between the legs. Flea allergy dermatitis requires treatment by a veterinarian. Fleas are also the intermediate host for dog tapeworm species.

Ticks

Dogs are infested primarily by the brown dog tick, which seldom bites humans and carries no human disease, and the less common American dog tick, which bites humans and carries Rocky Mountain spotted fever.

Dogs pick up ticks from infested premises or by running through woods, fields, grass, bushes, damp areas, and sandy beaches. The ticks attach themselves to the dog's skin and feed on its blood. After ticks mate, the female remains attached for several days, sucking the dog's blood and enlarging up to ten times normal size; then drops off her host and moves to a quiet spot to lay eggs—1000 to 5000 at a time. The eggs hatch into larvae or "seed ticks" after an incubation period of 3 to 8 weeks, depending on temperature and humidity. The seed ticks molt into nymphs and they, in turn, molt into adults, completing the life cycle.

When a tick bites a dog, it forces its barbed mouth parts deep into the dog's skin. The barbed mouth means the tick is not easy to pull out. Tick bites are painful and very irritating to dogs. The irritation leads to intense itching and persistent scratching, which often results in secondary skin infections. Ticks can cause anemia quickly because they ingest so much of the dog's blood.

To remove ticks that are present on the dog:

1. Examine the dog's body thoroughly to locate all ticks. Check inside the ears, between the feet, under the front legs—areas ticks hide in.

2. Soak the ticks in alcohol or a small amount of tick spray. This will help paralyze and asphyxiate each tick and cause it to release its barbed-mouth grip.

3. Wood ticks and dog ticks must be removed and killed so that they will not spread Rocky Mountain spotted fever. (See also "External Parasites: Rocky Mountain Spotted Fever.") All parts of the tick should be pulled out; the tick should not be crushed and the person removing it should not touch it with bare hands.

4. Carefully grasp each tick with a tweezers or forceps. If you use your fingers, shield your hand with a piece of paper or paper towel.

5. Do not twist the tick to remove it, but pull it straight outward. Be sure all the parts are removed and that the

head does not break off, remain in the dog's skin, and cause an infection.

6. After removing each tick, apply an antiseptic to the area.

7. As soon as the ticks have been removed from the dog, burn them or flush them down the toilet. Do not crush them.

8. Wash your hands thoroughly with soap and water.

Flea and Tick Control

Flea and tick control is done with several products and depends on the type of pet you own, the animal's environment, and your climate.

Flea and tick collars are effective for most dogs. They contain vaporizing agents that kill fleas or ticks for up to 4 months. Special collars are available for puppies and for large dogs. Observe the following rules when you use a flea or tick collar.

1. Before you purchase the collar, check for breed restrictions listed on the package. Certain types of collars should not be worn on Whippets and Greyhounds.

2. Read the manufacturer's directions carefully.

3. Remove the collar from its sealed envelope and allow it to air for 24 hours before putting it around the dog's neck.

4. When applying the collar, fasten it comfortably around your dog's neck. You should be able to slip two fingers between the collar and the animal's neck.

5. After the collar is applied, cut off any excess.

6. Remove the collar if it (or the dog) gets wet.

7. Remove the collar before using other flea and tick control products. Check with your veterinarian before you use a combination of flea/tick products, which can be hazardous.

8. Inspect the skin (especially around the neck) frequently for redness or other signs of irritation. Certain breeds may be hypersensitive to the chemicals contained in the flea or tick collars. If you see such a reaction, remove the collar immediately, and inform your veterinarian (if the irritation is severe).

9. Do not place a flea or tick collar on a dog that will be wormed or is scheduled to have surgery.

10. Do not place a flea or tick collar on a sick or debilitated dog.

11. While informing your veterinarian about any medical problem, mention it if the dog has been wearing a collar.

12. If you own a cat, do not place a dog flea collar on the cat.

Before you put on a collar, bathing your dog with insecticidal shampoo will help kill fleas and ticks. Many fine-quality, safe, nonirritating shampoos are formulated especially to rid puppies and adult dogs of fleas, lice, and ticks. When shampooing, allow the lather to remain on the coat for several minutes for the insecticide to take effect. An alternative is a flea/tick powder or spray, which is convenient for spot application if needed.

In severe cases of infestation, a flea and tick dip may be necessary. Control of the dog's environment is important to prevent reinfestation. Vacuum the dog's bedding, your furniture and rugs. After vacuuming, burn the vacuum bags to destroy all eggs and larvae. Clean the cracks in the floors and around the baseboard. Indoor insecticidal sprays can be applied directly to furniture, rugs, drapes, and the dog's bedding. For severe problems in a house or kennel, use a pressurized indoor fumigant fogger, which will penetrate deeply into hard-to-reach areas and is designed to be set off *after an area has been evacuated.* Be sure to read label directions carefully and stay out of the area for the required length of time. Lawn and kennel dusts and outdoor repellents are available to reduce the possibilities of your dog bringing parasites back into the house or kennel.

To learn more about which products and methods to use to control fleas and ticks, talk to your veterinarian.

Rocky Mountain Spotted Fever

Rocky Mountain spotted fever is transmissible to man by the American dog tick and the Rocky Mountain spotted fever or western wood tick. Ticks are oval-shaped blood-sucking parasites with eight legs sticking out from the sides of their bodies like those of a crab. Both ticks are brown; adult males have mottled white areas on their top sides, while adult females have a large white-to-cream shield on top immediately behind their heads. When an adult female is fully engorged, she becomes bluish and is about $1/2$ inch long.

The name "Rocky Mountain spotted fever" is somewhat misleading, because while the disease was discovered in the Rocky Mountains in the last half of the 19th century, today less than 6% of reported cases occur there. In the last decade, the disease has been reported in all of the United States except Alaska and Hawaii. It is a national problem with public health significance; the majority of its victims are children from ages 3 to 16 years.

The disease is difficult to diagnose because its early symptoms are not unusual. The first signs are sudden headache, overall discomfort, fever, loss of appetite, muscle aches, eye pains, and sensitivity to light. More specific symptoms appear a few days later: higher temperature, often as high as 104°F (40°C), swelling of the tissues, and a hemorrhaging rash which appears on the feet and ankles and then spreads to the hands and other parts of the body. At first the rash is flat and bright red, almost like a measles rash, but it quickly becomes dark red and raised.

If you or your children are bitten by a tick, have removed ticks from your dog, or live in a tick-infested area, and you develop these symptoms, contact your physician immediately. When Rocky Mountain spotted fever is diagnosed *promptly* and treated with the correct antibiotics, it can be cured completely. If the disease is not treated, it can be fatal or can damage vital organs permanently.

How can you best protect your family from Rocky Mountain spotted fever?

1. Keep pets and living quarters as tick free as possible. Examine every pet often (especially around the ears and between the toes) to avoid heavy infestation. Check with a veterinarian or pest exterminator about necessary tick control measures for your pets, home, and yard.

2. If you live, work, hike, camp or if your children play in a tick-infested area, apply a repellent containing DEET —diethylmeta-toluamide—to skin and clothing. Be sure the repellent is applied around any openings in clothing, such as collars, pants legs/cuffs, waistbands, belts, buttons, and zippers, and especially around sock tops.

3. Examine family members regularly for the presence

of ticks. You seldom feel ticks crawling or biting, so they can become attached and feed for days before being noticed. Ticks like warm, moist areas: check the scalp, behind the ears, in the armpits, under breasts, around the waist, the groin area, the soles of the feet, and between the toes. Remove ticks as soon as they are discovered, using the same methods previously described for removing ticks from dogs.

Lice

Lice, which are less common than fleas and ticks, are tiny, pale parasites which are spread by direct contact. Dogs can be infested with sucking or biting lice. Lice are hard to see, especially on long-coated dogs, since they are less than 1/10 inch long. Biting lice move slowly through the hair, while sucking lice attach themselves to the dog's skin and feed. Lice can be found all over the dog's body; sucking lice are found most often around the ears and the back of the neck.

Lice complete their life cycle on the dog. Adult females produce a number of eggs or "nits" which are pale and transparent and stick to the dog's hair. The eggs hatch and become adults in 3 to 4 weeks, depending on temperature. Lice also carry dog tapeworm species.

Symptoms of lice include intense itching, scratching, and biting of infested areas and loss of hair. If neglected and allowed to become heavily infested, a dog with sucking lice can develop anemia rapidly.

To remove lice, use a shampoo or dip effective against fleas and ticks. The treatment may have to be repeated after several weeks to destroy new lice that have developed from eggs. To get more effective results it is advisable to clip the hair from long-coated dogs before shampooing or dipping. Although lice complete their life cycle on the dog, the bedding and surrounding areas should be vacuumed and sprayed as an extra precaution to prevent reinfestation. Consult your veterinarian if the infestation is severe.

Mites

Members of the mite order cause many skin problems. Most mites are microscopic, that is, not visible to the eye.

To determine their presence your veterinarian will take a scraping of the upper layer of the dog's skin for examination. The skin problems caused by mites are generally known as mange. It is important to identify species of mite before treatment begins.

Some of the common mites we will discuss are ear mites, sarcoptic and demodectic mange mites, and cheyletiella mites.

Ear Mites

Ear mites are more common in cats, but also occur in dogs. *Otodectes cynotis* is transmitted by direct contact and completes its life cycle in the host's ear. The mites live on the skin surface of the ear and ear canal, where they bite the skin and feed on lymph. They are not visible to the naked eye but can be suspected when a dog shakes its head violently or constantly scratches or rubs its ears. The earflaps and edges and insides of the ears may be swollen and irritated and you may see dark brown, foul-smelling fragments inside the ear. Secondary ear infections and even hematoma can occur from the frequent shaking and rubbing of an infested dog.

If you own a magnifying glass, you can see ear mites. Remove some waxy fragments and place them on a black background or a piece of glass. Through the magnifying glass the mites look like tiny white moving specks.

Your veterinarian can confirm the presence of ear mites by microscopic examination. Once the mite is identified, it is best to let your veterinarian give the first treatment, removing all fragments from the ear and applying an oil-based solution containing an insecticide. Treatment continues at home and depends on the product prescribed. During home treatment, the dog should be isolated from additional sources of infection. The premises should be sprayed with insecticide.

Sarcoptic Mange Mites

The sarcoptic mange mite, or *Sarcoptes scabiei canis,* causes sarcoptic mange or scabies. The disease is spread by direct contact, as the mite completes its life cycle in 10 to 14 days on its host. Mating takes place on the skin surface; then the female mites burrow into the dog's skin, which causes intense itching, and form tunnels where their eggs are laid. In 3 to 8 days the eggs hatch in the tunnels and the larvae migrate to the skin, molt into a nymph stage, and then become adults.

Sarcoptic mange is signaled by intense itching. A small scale formation develops on various parts of the dog's body, usually the ear tips, head, elbows, hocks, and underside of the tail. In advanced cases, the mange may extend over the entire body surface and the skin will appear dry, thickened, and wrinkled. The dog may scratch constantly, lose its appetite, and become generally weak.

Sarcoptic mange is extremely contagious; it spreads rapidly from dog to dog and can infect humans. Diagnosis is made by skin scraping. Treatment generally consists of bathing with an antiseborrheic shampoo to remove the scales, followed by insecticidal dips at intervals that depend on the product used. Since sarcoptic mange is contagious, all pets in the family should be treated at the same time. The premises should be sprayed with an insecticide.

Demodectic Mange Mites

The demodectic mange mite, or *Demodex canis,* is a tiny cigar-shaped parasite, also called the follicular or red mange mite. It is thought to be present in the hair follicles (and occasionally, sebaceous glands) of most dogs, though not all of them develop lesions. It is not known why some dogs develop demodectic mange and others do not, but it is thought that demodectic mange is associated with periods of stress. The mites can be found in the sebaceous glands around a bitch's nipples; her puppies can become infected while nursing. Some dogs can be carriers; although not exhibiting signs of the disease, bitches can have litters affected with demodectic mange.

Demodectic mange occurs in two forms. In the squamous or localized form small, red, scaly areas are produced around the lips, mouth, eyes, ears or on or near the front legs, accompanied by loss of hair. In the pustular or generalized form the condition becomes more advanced, with extensive loss of hair and thickened, crusty, reddened skin over large parts of the body surface. The dog scratches almost constantly and the skin has a tendency to crack and bleed, with a rancid smell, usually the result of bacterial infection.

Both forms of demodectic mange require immediate attention. Diagnosis is made by skin scraping. Most dogs with a localized infestation can be treated with any of a number of effective products. When treatment is successful, the hair should start growing back in about 2 weeks and the dog should be completely recovered after 10 weeks. Along with the treatment, the dog should have a well-balanced diet and not be subjected to periods of stress. Treatment of the generalized form takes much longer and the prognosis is poor; it is important to identify any bacterial infections and treat them with appropriate antibiotics.

Cheyletiella Mites

The cheyletiella mite is large and nonburrowing; it lives on the skin surface and is spread by direct contact. *Cheyletiella yasguri* is more common than *C. parasitavorax;* both complete their life cycles on the host. Puppies seem to be the most susceptible dogs. Symptoms include mild itching with profuse yellowish gray scales resembling dandruff, especially on the back, croup, and top of the head.

Treatment includes cleaning with an antiseborrheic shampoo to remove the scales and insecticidal dips at intervals that depend on the product used. Every pet in your household must be treated. The premises should be cleaned and treated with insecticidal sprays and all pet bedding should be laundered thoroughly and sprayed.

SKIN PROBLEMS

Clean, healthy, supple skin is important for every dog. Skin disease is a real problem for the dog owner, as nothing is more frustrating than watching a dog constantly lick or scratch itself. Often the dog's furious scratching or rubbing aggravates the condition and exposes the pet to secondary infection.

Skin problems in dogs are as varied as those in humans. In addition to external parasites, there are allergies, acne, fungus infections, ringworm, hot spots, eczema, and seborrhea. It's best to consult your veterinarian at the first sign of any dermatological problem. Correct diagnosis is necessary for proper treatment. *Do not attempt home treatment. Skin conditions can be aggravated and made worse by choice of incorrect preparations.* Skin allergies may be caused by food, weed/tree pollens, grass, dust, or bites from fleas and mites. (See "Allergy/Allergic Reactions" in section I.) Some other common skin problems follow.

Acne

Canine acne, caused by an inflammation of the sebaceous glands, is seen mostly in dogs 3 to 12 months of age; it often heals naturally as the dog matures. Symptoms include red and/or pus-filled bumps on the chin and lips, or occasionally on the back of the neck and lower abdomen. The condition can usually be cleared up by washing affected areas daily with an antibacterial shampoo such as pHisoHex® (available by prescription), but severe cases may require antibiotic treatment.

Ringworm

Ringworm is a skin infection that is frequently confused with mange; it is not caused by a parasite but by a fungus. (There is no "worm" involved.) The infection starts in the horny outer layer of the dog's skin, where the fungi develop from spores. They grow partly down the hair follicle and enter the hairs. The disease gets its name because the affected areas assume a circular shape. Variations are seen, however, and the lesions can be oval or irregularly shaped. Ringworm can be transmitted from animal to animal and from soil to animal; certain types are transmissible to man.

Symptoms include circular or irregular patches on the face, body, or legs. Some lesions can hardly be seen;

312

others may be scaly patches or crusted formations, with hair loss. The fungal elements can cause secondary bacterial infections under the crusts.

If you suspect ringworm, the dog should be taken immediately to a veterinarian where diagnosis will be made by microscopic examination with a Wood's light or by culturing the fungus. Treatment includes clipping off the infected hair and applying fungicidal ointments or dips. Your veterinarian also may prescribe Griseofulvin, a drug which stops fungi from growing in the hair follicle. Treatment may take several weeks to several months. During recovery, remember to destroy any scaly matter or hair that falls off the dog. After handling the dog, wash your hands with an antibacterial soap, such as pHisoHex® (available by prescription), before touching any parts of your body.

The dog's living area should be cleaned and all bedding, combs, brushes, and other contaminated items should be washed and sterilized in a Clorox solution (1 part Clorox to 8 parts water) or replaced. To avoid contamination of others, affected dogs should be isolated from people and other pets.

Eczema and Hot Spots

Eczema is common among smooth and long-coated dogs. It can be the result of allergies, external parasites, dietary deficiencies, hormone imbalances, neglect in grooming, or predisposition. Dogs do not inherit eczema, but certain strains in every breed seem more inclined to develop it.

In dry eczema the skin looks scaly, with cracked and inflamed spots which the dog scratches constantly; in moist eczema or "hot spots" red, moist, ulcerated spots develop in the skin and are made worse by the dog's biting and scratching. Both types occur in purebreds and mixed breeds at any season, but most often in damp, warm climates. Canine eczema is not transmissible to humans.

Eczema appears suddenly, and if it remains untreated, it can make a dog miserable. Because the affected areas are so itchy, the dog's constant licking, scratching, and biting causes additional irritation and damage. Treatment

313

should be prescribed by a veterinarian. A number of lotions provide temporary relief, but eczema must also be treated internally in most cases.

Seborrhea

Seborrhea is a common skin problem of dogs, often seen in Cocker and Springer Spaniels, Schnauzers, and German Shepherds. Three types of seborrhea can occur:

1. Seborrhea sicca, commonly known as dandruff, is distinguished by dry, grayish white scales interspersed through the dog's hair.

2. Seborrhea oleosa is distinguished by greasy specks which cling to the dog's hairs and look like lice "nits." Some of the coat and skin is covered with greasy particles and yellowish scales. Dogs with oily seborrhea often have a rancid or greasy odor.

3. In seborrhea dermatitis the scaliness or greasiness is accompanied by hair loss, redness, and itching.

Since its cause is unknown, seborrhea can be controlled but not cured. It usually responds favorably to treatment, but tends to recur. Treatment includes bathing with an antiseborrheic shampoo such as Seleen®, Sebafon®, or Thiomar® at intervals that depend on the severity of the condition, plus application of ointments to reduce scale and crust formation. If the dog is scratching constantly, your veterinarian may prescribe corticosteroids to relieve itching.

GROOMING

Whether your dog is a purebred or a mixed-breed, and whether its coat is short or long, its hair must be cared for regularly. Regular grooming is important not only to make a dog look better, but also for its physical health and mental fitness. Dogs seem to be happier and more content when they look their best, and most dog experts will agree that when a dog is groomed regularly, it is less likely to suffer from common skin problems, excessive itching, shedding, and infestation by external parasites.

Different types of dog hair require different grooming procedures. Some dogs need only brushing and combing, while others need to be clipped, scissored, plucked, or stripped. Smooth-coated dogs are the easiest to groom. The best way to keep their coats in good condition is to brush regularly with a fine quality bristle brush or hound glove. Dogs with double-textured coats (a harsh outercoat and soft undercoat), such as the Collie, Siberian Husky, German Shepherd, Old English Sheepdog, and many mixed-breeds, do not require complicated grooming but do need regular brushing, especially during the late spring and early fall shedding periods when great amounts of dead hair are shed. Dogs with long coats that fall flat over the sides of the body to the ground should have their coats separated into sections and brushed in layers. Certain terriers and other wire-coated breeds are stripped or plucked. Poodles, Bedlington Terriers, Kerry Blue Terriers, and some other breeds require expert clipping and scissoring. Spaniels, Setters, and some other breeds are groomed with clippers and thinning shears.

If your dog's coat requires complicated grooming, you may want to have it done by a professional dog groomer or learn how to do it yourself. It can be time-consuming. Never clip, scissor, pluck, or strip your dog's coat unless you know how to do it correctly. If you wish to learn complicated grooming procedures, we recommend that you purchase a book that provides detailed grooming instructions for your breed and that you contact your groomer or grooming school to arrange for proper instruction.

Every dog needs to be brushed. Generally, the longer the hair, the more frequently it will need brushing. Smooth and double-coated breeds should be brushed about twice a week. Ideally, long-haired dogs should be brushed daily; however, a thorough brushing two or three times a week will keep the coat in good condition. Brushing a dog's hair achieves the following results:

1. Removes dirt, dust, and dead hair
2. Spreads the natural oils evenly throughout the coat
3. Massages the skin and helps stimulate new hair growth
4. Helps prevent tangles from forming
5. Helps keep the skin clean and free from irritation

All long-haired dogs should be brushed thoroughly from the skin out. On dogs with very long coats, try to part the hair to the skin, letting one hand hold down the unbrushed hair to separate it from the section being brushed. Use gentle strokes that do not pull out excess hair or scratch the dog's skin. After a thorough brushing, comb through the coat with a dog comb to be sure all tangles have been removed.

You will need the correct type of brush and comb, which, depending on your dog's coat, can be a bristle, pin, or wire brush and a fine-, medium-, or coarse-tooth comb. Ask your groomer or pet suppliers dealer to show you the right tools. You can match the brush and comb to your dog's coat type, making grooming easier for you and more comfortable for the dog.

Along with a brush and comb you will need a coat conditioner: a specially formulated product that is sprayed lightly onto the hair before brushing. It makes brushing easier, helps remove tangles, eliminates dryness, and adds a shine to the hair which deepens and enriches the natural coat color. Products which contain protein, such as Ring 5 Protein Coat Conditioner, will help repair damaged hair. If you neglect your dog's coat or brush incorrectly, especially in damp or humid climates, the coat can become tangled quickly. Large tangles are troublesome to remove, as no dog will sit quietly while you pull through its hair trying to remove mats. Special tangle-removing products are available that make mat removing easier and faster for you and more bearable for the dog. Coat conditioners and tangle removers can be purchased from your pet supplies dealer.

There are other grooming requirements besides brushing: bathing, drying, and care of the ears, eyes, and nails. If your dog is trimmed professionally, you can rely on your groomer to attend to these during the dog's regular appointments. If the dog does not go to a groomer, it is up to you.

Health Check

When you have established a regular brushing/combing routine, learn to use the sessions as a means of checking your dog's health. Periodic visual observations, especially if supplemented by manual inspections, can reveal health problems which, if diagnosed and treated promptly by a veterinarian, will save your dog much discomfort and suffering.

Each time you brush or comb your dog's coat, look for signs of fleas, ticks, or other external parasites and evidence of skin disease. Feel the dog's skin and coat. Is the skin supple or dry? Is the hair soft and shiny or brittle? Many factors can affect a dog's skin and coat temporarily, but when your dog has constant problems with excessive shedding, itching, a dull coat, or dry skin, it is time to seek your veterinarian's advice. Check any sudden loss of hair, inflamed areas, or signs of tenderness or lumps under the skin immediately with your veterinarian.

Take time to examine the inside of your dog's mouth. Foul breath or tartar at the gum line may indicate mouth disease. Early detection and prompt cleaning and care may prevent the disease from spreading to other areas of the body.

Check your dog's ears, nose, and eyes frequently. Is the dog holding one ear lower than the other, scratching, or shaking its head frequently? Do the ears have a foul smell? Ear mites or bacterial infection can be suspected. Are the eyes inflamed or running? Many canine diseases begin with a discharge from the eyes and nose.

Along with the visual and manual inspections at brushing time, it is important to notice changes in behavior or attitude that may indicate the beginning of disease. Changes in eating, drinking, or sleeping habits, or in bowel or bladder function, and unusual discharges from body openings should be reported to your veterinarian.

Bathing

How often you bathe your dog depends on breed, type of skin and hair, how quickly the dog gets dirty, and the temperature and humidity of your area. Most long-haired dogs are bathed monthly, while the harsh- and double-coated breeds seldom need a bath more than four times a year, since shampooing softens the coat texture. If you use a fine shampoo formulated for dogs, however, you can bathe them as often as necessary.

Where you bathe your dog depends on its size. Small

and medium-sized dogs will fit in one side of a laundry tub, but larger dogs usually will need to be shampooed in a bathtub. Before bathing it, brush and comb the dog thoroughly to be sure all tangles have been removed from its coat. To save a lot of aggravation, assemble all bathing supplies before you put the dog in the tub: a rubber bath mat for the tub bottom to keep the dog from slipping, a shower spray or rubber hose, shampoo, a small sponge or soft brush for scrubbing, cotton balls, and a supply of clean towels.

Always use a shampoo that has been correctly balanced for dogs, as the pH range for the dog's skin and hair is not the same as that of humans. The acidity or alkalinity of a product is measured by its pH, which is 7 for neutral, 0 to below 7 for acid, and above 7 to 14 for alkali. Human skin and hair are slightly acid, so that "acid-balanced" or "nonalkaline," shampoos are correctly pH-balanced for humans. Dogs' skin and hair, however, are slightly alkaline, calling for an alkaline shampoo to maintain your dog's skin and coat at their healthiest, strongest state. Manufacturers such as Ring 5, Lambert Kay, and Oster have formulated many fine all-purpose shampoos for dogs, as well as tearless shampoos, insecticidal and medicated shampoos, shampoos which add texture to the hair, and shampoos for special coat colors.

After the dog is brushed and all bath supplies are at hand, place a cotton ball in each ear to keep the water out. If you do not use a tearless shampoo, place a drop of mineral oil in each eye to prevent irritation. Stand the dog on the bath mat in the tub and turn on the warm water. Using the shower spray or hose, wet the dog thoroughly to the skin. If the dog is upset or frightened, pat it gently and talk to it reassuringly. Squeeze shampoo on the wet hair and work from front to back, lathering the head, neck, body, legs, and tail with the sponge or soft brush. Wash the face last, taking care not to get shampoo into the dog's eyes. Rinse well from head to tail; if the dog has long hair, shampoo a second time and rinse thoroughly from head to tail and down the legs, making sure that all traces of shampoo are out of the coat.

After rinsing, squeeze the water out of the hair and let the dog shake. Remove the cotton balls and dry the insides of the earflaps. Wrap the dog in a clean towel to absorb excess moisture and remove the dog from the tub. Keep changing the towels and rubbing the hair until it is dry, or use a hair dryer, pointing the nozzle at a section of wet hair, and at the same time brushing the hair from the skin out. In cold weather, keep your dog indoors 4 to 6 hours after a bath.

Summer Care

Many a dog suffers needlessly in summer because of its owner's thoughtlessness. Remember, when you are uncomfortable from the heat, your dog probably is too. Here are some summer hazards of which the pet owner should be aware:

1. Provide plenty of clean, fresh drinking water at all times. Too little water can cause dehydration, even kidney problems.

2. If your dog is less active in summer, you may want to slightly reduce its food intake.

3. Pick up and clean food pans promptly. This helps keep insects away and keeps your dog from eating spoiled food.

4. Strenuous activities or exercise should be scheduled for early morning or early evening, and never when the sun is high.

5. Shade is imperative for outdoor dogs. Cool, shaded areas should be available for protection from direct sunlight.

6. Keep the dog's kennel run or outdoor area clean. Infestation by fleas, ticks, and other external parasites can cause serious problems in hot weather. Learn how to rid your dog of external parasites and how to prevent reinfestation.

7. Learn how to prevent heatstroke. (See "Heatstroke" in section I.) Many dogs die every summer because of owners' carelessness about heatstroke. Learn the symptoms, the necessary emergency action, and especially how to prevent it.

8. Regular grooming and coat care are necessary for all breeds in hot weather. If you cannot spend extra time on a long-haired dog, ask your groomer to select a short and attractive pet trim which will keep it cooler and more comfortable.

319

9. Each time you brush your dog, check the rear end and remove any soiled or matted clumps of hair. Keep the hindquarters clean to prevent flies from biting the dog.

10. Each time you brush the dog, examine the skin for external parasites.

11. Inspect the feet regularly. Make sure the hair between the pads is trimmed short to keep summer irritations from starting.

12. Remember that hot weather, direct sunlight, and warm winds dry out the dog's coat just as they do your own hair. Use a coat conditioner to help keep the dog's skin soft and the hair shiny, and to eliminate dryness.

13. Hot weather and high humidity can cause problems for the double-coated breeds which shed much of their undercoats in late spring and early summer. Owners are sometimes confused and believe the dog should be clipped close for comfort. Fortunately, this incorrect practice is being abandoned. The combination of a harsh outer coat and soft undercoat holds back the sun's rays and acts as insulation. Regular brushing is necessary, however, as heat and high humidity can quickly mat the undercoat and cause skin problems.

Winter Care: Indoor Dogs

1. Every dog, smooth or long-coated, should be brushed and combed regularly. Remember that the warm, dry atmosphere of a house or apartment in winter can dry the skin and hair. It may be necessary to use a coat conditioner several times a week to keep the coat lustrous and to help lubricate the skin.

2. Make sure the dog is eating a well-balanced diet.

3. If your dog is groomed professionally every few weeks, ask your groomer to leave the hair slightly longer.

4. Dog coats and sweaters are a matter of preference and depend on how cold it gets in your area and your dog's activities outdoors. While some indoor dogs will not need a covering if they are active when outdoors:

    a. A coat or sweater is necessary for any smooth-coated dog when it will be outdoors for any length of time, especially if it will be inactive.

    b. After bathing or grooming (especially if the hair has been shortened), the dog should wear a sweater or coat when it goes outside.

5. If you bathe your dog at home, keep it indoors 4 to 6 hours afterward.

6. When a long-haired dog becomes soaked with snow or icy water after outdoor exercise, as soon as the dog comes indoors towel the hair to remove excess moisture, then brush and dry the hair thoroughly. This will keep mats and tangles from forming.

7. Avoid extreme changes in temperature. Do not keep the dog outside during the day and inside during the night or vice versa. Frequent extreme temperature changes can result in a sick dog.

8. The feet need special attention in winter. (See "Care of the Feet: Cold Weather Care.")

Winter Care: Outdoor Dogs

Dogs can be maintained outdoors during the winter if they are conditioned to exposure to the cold.

1. Outdoor dogs require more food in winter. They use up a lot of body energy to keep warm.

2. A kennel should be maintained at an even temperature. Avoid frequent and extreme temperature changes.

3. Kennel dogs should have sleeping quarters that are draft-free. If your kennels are unheated, be sure that drafts from doors and windows will not cause chilling.

4. If your kennels are heated, be sure all heating and electrical equipment is in good working order so there is no danger of fire.

5. Outside kennel runs should contain wooden platforms built off the ground for the dog to sit on.

6. If the dog lives in an outside house, be sure the structure is waterproof, draft-free, and raised off the ground to keep the floor from getting damp. Be sure the entrance to the house faces away from the wind. Provide a swinging door or hang a waterproof covering over the entrance (but be sure the dog can enter and leave its house without difficulty) to keep out drafts, rain, and snow. Inside the house, provide clean and warm bedding (blankets, cedar shavings, etc.) that the dog can snuggle into and become comfortable. Check the dog's water pan several times a day to be sure it hasn't frozen. When the temperature drops to near zero, consider bringing your dog inside to a warm, dry basement.

7. Every outdoor dog should be brushed and combed regularly. A dog with a well-brushed coat can withstand the cold better than one that is a mass of tangles and dead hair.

The Ears

Check your dog's ears regularly. Both short- and long-haired dogs experience ear problems; some breeds are more susceptible than others. Dogs with pendulous ears, such as Spaniels, Setters, and certain Hounds, are prone to ear troubles because there is little circulation around the ears. Poodles, Bedlington Terriers, Bichons Frises, and certain other breeds have hair growing inside their ears which needs to be pulled out periodically. If their hair is neglected and allowed to grow long inside the ear, wax and dirt will cling to it, causing air circulation to be cut off and resulting in infection. Breeds with erect ears may be subject to problems around the ear rims, but rarely suffering from internal infections.

How can you tell when your dog is having ear problems? You'd have to be uncaring not to notice! Usually the dog will scratch, sometimes so persistently that the earflaps bleed or a hematoma (a blood-filled blister that makes the earflap swell) develops. The dog may shake its head violently or rub its ear on the floor. The ears may be red and inflamed and there may be large amounts of dark brown, gummy, foul-smelling wax in the ears. An ear infection can cause the dog to lose its sense of balance; it will often hold the infected ear lower than the other. Often just touching the ear or putting a collar around the dog's neck causes it great pain and the dog may become irritable and snappy.

Such symptoms result from accumulation of dirt and wax, infestation by ear mites or ticks, foreign objects in the ear, or bacterial infections. It is wise to seek professional advice immediately. Don't delay: neglect of something minor can lead to a more serious condition. There is no one cure for all ear problems, so let your veterinarian diagnose the condition and prescribe appropriate treatment.

Cleaning the Ears

Regular cleaning of your dog's ears will result in a healthier, happier pet and will let you detect the beginning of troublesome ear conditions. How often the ears need to be cleaned depends on whether your dog is smooth or long-haired and whether it has erect or hanging ears. Cleaning once a month will keep the ears in good condition, but long-haired dogs with hanging ears may need more frequent attention. Use this step-by-step procedure to clean the ears:

1. Long-haired dogs with hanging ears should have the excess hair leading into the ear canal removed before cleaning. Sit your dog on a firm surface. Have an assistant restrain the dog if necessary. (See "Handling and Restraint" in section I.)

2. Turn the earflap backward. Use your thumb and index finger to carefully pull out any excess hair leading into the canal. Pull only a few hairs at a time; otherwise it will hurt the dog. It is not necessary to remove every hair, just enough to let the air circulate.

3. After excess hair has been removed, moisten a cotton ball with an ear lotion (available from your veterinarian or pet store, and formulated to clean the ears and help loosen excess wax accumulation). Carefully wipe the earflap and opening into the canal as far as you can see. Do not probe deep into the canal. If there is no evidence of wax accumulation or foul smell, a light swabbing is enough.

4. Should you notice a wax accumulation inside the ear, grasp the cartilage at the base of the ear (the projection covered by skin on both sides, immediately at the opening into the canal) and pull it gently outward and away from the head. Place several drops of ear lotion in the canal. When the ear is held open in this position, any liquid placed inside will make its way down the canal and promote proper cleaning.

5. Steady the head with one hand to keep the dog from shaking; use the other hand to massage the base of the ear to distribute the lotion inside.

6. Release your hold on the dog's muzzle after several seconds of massaging. As soon as you let go of the muzzle the dog probably will shake its head. Don't be

323

alarmed: this is nature's way of protecting the delicate structure of the ear canal and will help bring the wax to the surface.

7. Using a wax-softening lotion and massaging the base of the dog's ear will encourage accumulated wax to float to the surface. Once the wax is brought up, use clean cotton balls or Q-Tips to wipe out the ear until it is clean and dry. There is no need to probe deep into the ear to remove wax!

If you do not wish to clean your dog's ears yourself, let your veterinarian or groomer do the job, but the ears should not be neglected.

The Eyes

All dogs need regular eye care. The eyes should be checked daily and wiped free of any mucus and foreign matter that has collected on the inside corners. The best way is to saturate a cotton ball with warm water, raise the dog's head, gently open the lower lid, and allow the water to drop into the eye. Use dry cotton to absorb excess moisture or matter that floats to the eye corners. Do not rub over the eye with cotton. As our atmosphere becomes more polluted, remember that when you are affected by foreign matter in the air, your pet can also be bothered. A little extra care on your part can help to prevent minor irritations that may lead to serious problems.

Besides cleaning, coated dogs need regular facial grooming to help prevent eye irritation. Hair that comes in contact with the eyes can cause serious problems. The Old English Sheepdog, Puli, Briard, certain mixed breeds and other dogs with an abundance of facial hair, should be able to see through the thick coat which falls forward over the eyes. Comb their long hair above the eyes backward toward the base of the skull. Part a small section of hair about $1/2$ to 1 inch above each eye and comb it forward. Scissor each section to a length of $1/2$ to $3/4$ inch to form a sort of eyebrow above each eye. Now comb the rest of the long hair above the eyes forward again. The "eyebrows" will help keep the long hair out of the eyes.

Breeds such as Pekingese, Pugs, English Toy Spaniels, Japanese Chins, and Brussels Griffons have large, round, prominent eyes set in shallow sockets which can be scratched and irritated easily. If there are wispy hairs curling into the eyes and causing irritation, they should be plucked out carefully with your thumb and index finger—never trim them with scissors. Pekingese, Pugs, and Oriental Spaniels have facial wrinkles near the eyes which need regular attention. After cleaning the eyes, press the wrinkle away from the eyeball with your finger, then wash the skin with a cotton ball moistened with warm water. Dry with a tissue or cotton, then dip a Q-Tip in some cornstarch and lightly powder the wrinkled skin to keep it dry.

Terriers and other wire-coated breeds may have facial hairs which curl into the eyes and cause irritation. Wispy ends can be plucked with thumb and index finger, but if the short hairs are part of the beard or eyebrows, use a bit of hair-styling gel to control them until they grow long enough to blend naturally into the longer hair.

Breeds such as Maltese, Shih Tzu, and Yorkshire Terriers whose forelocks are pulled up and fastened above the eyes need special attention too. The hair above the eyes should not be cut with scissors. When tying up the forelocks or topknot, it is important to fasten the hair so that it does not break off and fall into the eyes. Once the topknot is parted and ready to be put up, comb through the hair to be sure it is smooth and in place, then fasten with a plastic barrette or small latex orthodontal-type band. Do not use a heavy rubber band, which would put too much pressure on the hair and cause it to break. Once the topknot is fastened, be sure it is not too tight to pull the eyes or the skin on top of the head. If wispy ends slip out after fastening, use a bit of hair-styling gel to hold them in place.

White and light-colored dogs often have dark-stained hair under the eyes, caused by discharge from the tear ducts. Excessive tearing can result from hereditary traits, allergy, neglect in grooming the face, infection of the tear ducts, conjunctivitis, or teething. Your veterinarian may be able to determine the cause of excessive tearing and control it. Daily attention to the hair under the eyes is the best way to control the staining. If the dog is a Poodle, clip and remove the stained hair frequently; but if a dog does not have its face clipped during regular grooming, comb the stained hair frequently with a fine-tooth comb to remove accumulated matter. Clean the area with warm water and cotton, then dry thoroughly. Products, available at most pet stores to camouflage the hair stain, are penciled onto the stained areas, then blended into the hair with your fingers. Such products should not be used in the dog's eyes.

Regular inspection of your dog's eyes can help you notice potentially dangerous conditions at an early stage. Observations of abnormality or continued irritation should be reported to your veterinarian immediately. Ocular diseases and conditions that affect dogs include:

1. Conjunctivitis: An inflammation of the conjunctiva, the membrane that lines the lids and covers the white of the eyeball. Symptoms include redness and swelling of the conjunctiva, watery or pussy discharge from the eyes, sensitivity to light, and persistent rubbing of the eyes. If the dog rubs or scratches its eyes continuously, the conjunctiva will become more inflamed. Conjunctivitis can be caused by bacterial infection or irritation from chemicals and dust, or it may be a secondary symptom of infections such as distemper or hepatitis.

2. Entropion: A condition in which the eyelids roll inward, allowing the hair on the lids to contact and irritate the eye. It is seen frequently in Golden, Labrador, and Chesapeake Bay Retrievers and in Chow Chows.

3. Ectropion: The reverse of entropion. The lid drops away from the eye and the third eyelid or "haw" becomes prominent. Ectropion is seen frequently in Bulldogs, Basset Hounds, Bloodhounds, and St. Bernards. Both conditions—entropion and ectropion—can be corrected by surgery.

4. Glaucoma: A disease in which elevated pressure within the eye destroys the nerve fiber layers, causing permanent damage and eventual blindness. Glaucoma usually occurs in the dog's middle years, at ages 4 to 8. If detected early, glaucoma can be controlled by surgery so that the dog is kept free of chronic discomfort.

5. Cataract: An opacity of the lens of the eye. (It is not a "film" on the outside of the eye.) A cataract may progress and cause blindness or it may remain small and hardly impair the dog's vision. Causes of cataracts include heredity, old age, endocrine problems such as dia-

betes, and infectious disease. Breeds which are known to develop hereditary cataracts include Poodles, Cocker Spaniels, Miniature Schnauzers, Boston Terriers, Fox Terriers, Afghan Hounds, Beagles, and Golden Retrievers. Many people believe cataracts occur most often in older days, but they can develop as early as birth in certain breeds. Juvenile or mature cataracts can be removed surgically with varying degrees of visual improvement.

6. Progressive retinal atrophy (PRA): A hereditary degeneration of the retina that eventually results in blindness. Progressive retinal atrophy occurs mostly in Poodles, Norwegian Elkhounds, Irish Setters, American and English Cocker Spaniels, all types of Retrievers, Shetland Sheepdogs, and Collies. The age at which PRA affects dogs varies with the breed. For instance, Irish Setters show symptoms of blindness at 6 months to 1 year of age; Norwegian Elkhounds at 2 to 3 years; and Poodles at 4 to 8 years. The most common symptom of PRA in all breeds is night blindness.

Because the eyes are fragile and sensitive organs, neglect of minor irritations can lead to serious problems. Any irritation that does not clear up within 24 hours or any abnormal condition should be reported to your veterinarian. Don't use ophthalmic ointments that were prescribed for a previous condition!

Readers with questions about ophthalmic care or problems may write to the Foundation for Veterinary Ophthalmology, 6223 Richmond Highway, Alexandria, VA 22303, a charitable organization established to raise and provide money for training and research in veterinary ophthalmology.

The Nose

Problems involving the exterior of the dog's nose are not too common. They may include sores, raw skin, or scabs, all caused by the dog rubbing its nose on wire (kennel runs, fences, etc.) or using its nose to dig. Application of an antiseptic skin cream usually will heal the nose quickly. Any irritation on the outside of the nose that does not heal promptly should receive veterinary attention. (For emergency problems involving the inside of the nose, see "Face and Neck Emergencies: Nosebleed" in section I.)

CARE OF THE FEET

Foot care, an important part of a dog's health care, is often neglected. Most dogs detest having their feet handled, so you should train your dog at an early age to allow its nails to be trimmed and its feet to be examined for potential problems. If you don't, a battle may take place each time you attempt to attend to the dog's feet.

The Nails

A dog's nails should be kept short. Excessively long nails can make the pet uncomfortable and cause serious damage to the feet, making walking and running painful, and in extreme cases of neglect, laming the dog.

It's surprising how many pet owners believe that dogs naturally wear down their nails. Especially with breeds that have an abundance of hair on their feet, most owners have no idea that potential problems are developing. Wild animals may wear down their nails in the course of daily activities, but usually not with house pets: the dogs that walk or exercise regularly on concrete or hard ground are in the minority. The average pet spends most of its time indoors, and even when it goes outside, generally it's to a grassy lawn or other surface too soft to keep the nails short.

Establish a regular schedule for nail trimming. The nails can be trimmed by a veterinarian or groomer, or you can learn to trim them yourself. The tools are a trimmer to shorten the nails and a file or emery board to smooth away rough edges. Always use a nail trimmer designed especially for dogs. There are two popular types—scissor and guillotine—and there are styles made especially for large breeds with heavier nails. Ask your pet supplies dealer to demonstrate nail trimmers, and decide which type is best for you and your breed. Most dogs eventually learn to accept having their nails trimmed without the need of restraint.

How to Trim the Nails

1. Sit the dog on a sturdy surface, facing you. It's important to keep the paw from shaking or moving, so have

someone restrain the dog, if necessary. (See "Handling and Restraint" in section I.)

2. Grasp one of the dog's feet in your hand and pull it slightly forward.

3. Hold the nail trimmer in your other hand. Insert the tip of the nail into the trimmer opening and cut each nail back a little at a time. The outside of the nail is made of a rather hard, horny protein called keratin. Inside the nail is a soft, fleshy area called the quick which contains the nerves and blood supply. Do not cut into the quick or you may sever the capillaries and cause bleeding. The quick usually can be seen inside the nail on white and light-colored dogs, but it is almost impossible to locate on dark-colored dogs. The tip of the nail grows downward, so a good rule to use in trimming dark nails is to cut them just behind the point where they begin to curve downward. If you are unsure at first, cut a little at a time and you will not seriously injure the nail.

4. Don't panic if you do cut into the quick and the nail bleeds. Press a styptic pencil or nail-clotting powder (available at pet stores) against the nail for a few seconds to stop the bleeding. If the bleeding continues, consult your veterinarian.

5. Your dog may have an extra toe on the inside of each front leg just above the paw. It is called a dewclaw: its attached nail should be trimmed like the others. Many breeds have their dewclaws removed several days after birth.

6. After all the nails have been trimmed, smooth away any rough edges with a nail file or emery board. This is especially important for Pugs, Pekingese, Bulldogs, and other breeds with large, round eyes set in shallow sockets. Should they attempt to scratch their faces, a ragged nail edge can scratch the eyes and cause serious problems.

Problems Caused by Overgrown Nails

The top of each nail grows in a curved downward direction, and in cases of extreme neglect the nails can grow backward in a semicircle and become attached to the foot pads. Also, neglected dewclaw nails can grow into the leg tissue. Both problems require immediate veterinary care.

Broken Toenails

Excessively long nails can not only cause damage to the feet, but become caught in fences and the like and break off. Often the break is not complete and the cracked nail remains partly attached to the toe. It is not a serious condition, but it can cause a lot of pain. Walking and running become uncomfortable, and in its efforts to compensate the dog may appear to be lame.

When a dog is troubled by a broken nail, try to remove it. If necessary, have someone restrain the pet (see "Handling and Restraint" in section I) as you take hold of the broken nail with your fingers or a tweezers and remove it with a swift, hard pull. There may be slight bleeding and a little pain when the nail is removed, but they usually subside quickly. If bleeding is severe, use a pressure bandage on the foot.

If removing the broken nail looks difficult, let your veterinarian do it. Special attention is necessary, if much tissue is exposed, to prevent infection that may require antibiotic treatment.

Interdigital Cysts

An interdigital cyst is a swelling or small abscess between the dog's toes. The swelling forms when the sweat glands between the toes become infected after a cut or scratch or when they are clogged by a mild dermatitis. Certain breeds—Bulldogs, Pekingese, and Scottish, Sealyham, and West Highland White Terriers—seem predisposed to develop interdigital cysts. More than one swelling may develop in a short time and both feet may be affected. If the swelling does not receive prompt attention, it may become abscessed.

An interdigital cyst is hot and red at first. The dog spends a lot of time licking the cyst without satisfaction. Eventually the swelling forces the toes apart and causes pressure on the cyst, which can be very painful when the dog walks. The cyst may burst and discharge pus; then the area may heal or it may form a thickening which from time to time exudes a purulent discharge.

Soak the affected foot in a quart of warm water into which 1 tablespoon of salt, Epsom Salts, or Massengill douche powder has been added. Repeat the soaks four times a day and dry the foot thoroughly after each soak. The soaks should help to draw the swelling to a head. You may occasionally apply a slight pressure to the cyst to encourage it to break and discharge its contents.

Some interdigital cysts are caused by staphylococcal or streptococcal infections and require veterinary treatment. The cyst may have to be lanced. Once the infectious agent is identified, the veterinarian will prescribe an appropriate antibiotic. He or she may have to bandage the feet to prevent licking until the infection has healed. If interdigital cysts are left untreated, surgical removal may be necessary. Preventive measures are important for dogs that are predisposed to develop these cysts. Cysts are less likely to develop if the hair between the toes and pads on the underside of each foot is clipped or trimmed short. Don't allow dirt to accumulate between the toes or foot pads. Wash the feet often, especially after the dog comes indoors after exercise in foul weather.

Cold Weather Care

Your dog's feet need special attention in snow and icy weather, especially if nearby streets are spread with rock salt to keep cars from slipping. Should some of the rock salt crystals collect between the dog's foot pads, the defrosting elements can cause burning and irritation.

Check the feet as soon as your dog comes indoors. Spread the toes and check between the pads on the underside of each foot. Remove any foreign matter immediately. Don't allow the dog to lick its pads: the defrosting elements can burn and irritate the tongue. Bathe the foot in warm water, dry thoroughly, then spread a thin layer of antiseptic ointment between the pads.

Other Problems

Chewing gum between toes: When dogs and children play together, it's not uncommon for chewing gum to find its way into hair between the pet's toes. The best way to remove it is to rub peanut butter into it. Let the peanut butter stand for a few minutes, then comb or work it out of the feet with your fingers. If you rub an ice cube over the gum it will soon become brittle and easy to pull out.

331

Tar in feet: Rub butter, margarine, or shortening into the tarred areas and let it remain between the toes until the tar softens and can be removed. Or you can soak the tarred area in warm water, then in mineral oil. Repeat until the tar loosens and can be worked out from between the toes. Wash and rinse the feet thoroughly.

CARE OF THE MOUTH

Baby or Deciduous Teeth

Begin paying attention to your dog's teeth and mouth during puppyhood. The "baby" or deciduous teeth begin to break through the gums at age 3 weeks. Baby teeth are softer, thinner, and more pointed than permanent teeth. By the time the puppy is 6 weeks of age, all 28 temporary teeth are usually in place.

The Teething Process

Between 12 to 14 weeks of age, the puppy's baby teeth begin to loosen and fall out as the permanent teeth start coming in. With exception of the canines (the four tusk-like teeth—one in each quadrant), the baby teeth are loosened by pressure from the permanent teeth growing underneath. The permanent canines can erupt through the gums beside the baby canines, with both teeth remaining in the gums for several months.

During teething, the puppy's mouth should be checked regularly to see that the deciduous teeth are coming out without problems. Check the canines for double teeth, and if there are any, advise your veterinarian, who may wish to pull the temporary canine to avoid serious problems in tooth alignment and adult bite.

The teething period is painful for many young dogs, which often develop a slight fever from teething.

Toys During the Teething Process

If a puppy has swollen and irritated gums it acts much like a teething baby, trying to put anything available into its mouth for relief. Give the puppy safe things to chew on; they help loosen the baby teeth as well as relieve the irritation of sore gums. Rawhide chips, bones, and chew twists, hard rubber balls and rings, and nylon bones are welcomed by the puppy at this time—not to mention that they save your furniture, rugs, and shoes from being chewed up. Do not give a puppy a toy that can be swallowed whole or torn apart into small pieces and swallowed, possibly causing intestinal obstruction. Noise-makers on squeaky toys should be nonremovable—otherwise, remove them. Avoid toys stuffed with sawdust or pellets if they can be torn apart easily.

A cold knucklebone (one that cannot splinter) will help soothe the irritated gums, but *never give chicken, steak, chop, or rib bones to a dog, as sharp pieces can become lodged in the throat or pierce the intestinal wall.* Remember: Chewing is important during the teething period because it helps loosen the baby teeth and aids normal jaw development.

Permanent Teeth

The permanent teeth are usually in place by 6 months of age. The normal number is 42 (20 in the upper jaw and 22 in the lower jaw); some breeds may have a jaw structure that does not have space for 42 teeth. Either some of the teeth will be missing or there will be an irregular bite caused by the pressure of one tooth on another.

Importance of Immunization and Nutrition During Puppyhood

During puppyhood, diet and immunization are important to dental health. Disease or nutritional deficiencies can permanently damage the tooth enamel. The elevated temperature during distemper or antibiotics used to treat the disease may cause the enamel of the permanent teeth to become pitted and yellow. Antibiotic discoloration may be temporary, affecting only the baby teeth, or may be permanent. Hepatitis and leptospirosis can affect the development of tooth enamel. Your puppy should eat a well-balanced diet and be vaccinated for distemper, hepatitis, and leptospirosis at the proper time.

333

Care of the Teeth

Proper nutrition and home dental care combined with regular veterinary checkups contribute to good teeth in the mature dog. Clean teeth and healthy gums are important to a dog's general health. Have the dog's teeth examined by a veterinarian semiannually and cleaned if necessary.

Dental Plaque and Bad Breath

Between professional checkups, a dog's teeth should be checked and cleaned regularly at home. The object of home care is to control dental plaque, a sticky, invisible film consisting of food particles, saliva, and bacteria which clings to the teeth. Plaque which collects between the teeth and around the gum line will build up if not removed soon after forming, and eventually the layers will mineralize into a hard, brown substance known as tartar or calculus. The high, alkaline pH level of canine saliva stimulates the conversion of dental plaque into tartar faster than in humans. The gums, irritated by the tartar buildup, become swollen and inflamed. The dog's breath becomes foul-smelling. If the condition is ignored, the irritation spreads to deeper tissues and the bone in which the teeth are embedded. Pockets form around the teeth and they loosen. Cavities in dogs are almost nonexistent, but if buildup of plaque and tartar remains untreated, a general infection can develop which may result in the loss of several teeth while the dog is young, or even in early death.

How to Clean the Teeth

The easiest way to prevent the buildup of dental plaque is to clean the teeth regularly with either of the following:

1. A flavored toothpaste for dogs which contains abrasive agents and is totally digestible (one brand, DVM, is available at most pet stores)
2. A mixture of equal parts baking soda and salt with a little water added to make a paste

Clean the teeth with a soft toothbrush or piece of gauze. A children's brush is recommended for small and medium

334

dogs, and a regular brush for large or giant breeds. Brush the teeth as you do your own: use gentle circular scrubbing strokes on each side and don't forget the biting surface of the back teeth. If your dog objects to a toothbrush, wrap a piece of soft gauze bandage around your index finger, squeeze on some toothpaste or dip into the soda/salt mixture, and rub gently over the teeth. After cleaning the teeth, rinse the dog's mouth with water. If your dog is trained from puppyhood to have its mouth opened and teeth examined, it will not object.

Other Mouth Odors

Certain breeds, sporting dogs and others with pendulous lips, sometimes have foul odors around the mouth even when the teeth are cleaned regularly. On each side of the dog's mouth there is a fold of skin in the lips. Some breeds have deeper folds and particles of food collect inside and cause irritation and a terrible odor. Sometimes this must be corrected surgically. If the lip fold is causing an odor problem, the area should be cleaned regularly.

Providing Safe Toys

A final word about toys. Make every effort to provide interesting, safe toys, which contribute greatly to the dog's mental and physical well-being. If you are away from home a great deal—especially if you have a job—and the dog is alone often, it may become discontented and destructive if it has nothing interesting to do.

NUTRITION

If you love your dog, you want to build a solid nutritional foundation to develop every potential of good bone structure and muscles, supple skin, shiny coat, bright eyes, and healthy teeth.

A dog should be fed a balanced diet containing correct proportions of protein, carbohydrates, fat, vitamins, minerals, and water. Good nutrition is essential at all ages, not only for growth, reproduction, and maintenance, but for optimum levels of activity and for repair of bodily damage and resistance to infection and other disease. To effectively sustain a dog, its food should:

1. Be agreeable to the dog, so that it is eaten in adequate amounts
2. Contain the minimum daily requirements for protein, carbohydrates, fat, vitamins, minerals, and water in a form that can be utilized by the dog
3. Supply enough energy to meet the dog's needs. Fat, carbohydrates, and proteins supply fuel necessary for body heat and activity. Energy requirements are affected by age, size, general condition, temperament, exercise, and environment, and can vary considerably even among dogs of the same breed. Sporting dogs used in the field require more calories than the same breeds as house pets. Dogs that live outdoors in cold weather need more energy than dogs that live indoors. Excitable and boisterous dogs need more energy than those that are quiet and well behaved. And on a per-pound basis, smaller breeds need more energy than larger dogs
4. Supply the necessary nutrients for the particular phase of the life cycle for which the food is being given

Essential Nutrients

Each nutrient has a definite purpose and relationship to the dog's body, and no one nutrient will maintain good health; all must be given in proper proportions. Specific amounts depend on age, size, environment, physical condition, and amount of exercise or activity.

Protein is one of the most important nutrients in a dog's diet for the growth and development of body tissues and for maintenance of optimum health. Often called "nature's building blocks," proteins are the nucleus of building material for the body organs, muscles, skin, coat, nails, and blood, and also are a source of heat and energy.

Protein is composed of smaller molecules known as amino acids; the number and sequence of amino acids in a protein determine its structure. The dog's body needs 23 amino acids, all but 10 of which can be synthesized in the body. These 10 are called essential amino acids because they must be furnished in the diet: arginine, histidine, isoleucine, leucine, lysine, methionine, phenyl-alanine, treonine, tryptophan, and valine. If one essential amino acid is lacking, even for a short time, protein synthesis will drop to an inadequate level.

Proteins are derived from plant and animal sources; nutritive value and digestibility depends on the source. Animal proteins are utilized more efficiently than plant proteins. Sources of high-quality animal proteins include meat, fish, poultry, milk, cheese, and eggs. The National Academy of Sciences, in *Nutrient Requirements of Dogs,* states that whole egg protein supplies nearly optimum concentrations of the amino acids needed by dogs. (When eggs are fed as a source of protein, they should be cooked, not raw. Raw eggs contain avidin, which couples with biotin—one of the B-complex vitamins—in the intestine, preventing its absorption.) Sources of plant proteins include soybeans, legumes, and grain products.

Carbohydrates supply energy for the dog's body and provide the bulk necessary for proper intestinal function. The main sources of carbohydrates in food are starches, sugars, and cellulose.

No specific requirements have been established, but dogs can utilize large amounts of carbohydrates in a well-balanced diet. Dog foods often contain a high level of carbohydrates because they are a low-priced source of nourishment. To make room for adequate amounts of protein and fat, animal nutritionists recommend that carbohydrates comprise a maximum of 65% of the dry weight of a dog's diet.

Fats supply essential fatty acids, are concentrated sources of energy, and add taste and texture to food. They also carry the fat-soluble vitamins—A, D, E, and K—within the body. Three fatty acids, linoleic, linolenic, and arachidonic, are defined as "essential" because the body cannot produce them. Linoleic acid is essential to maintain healthy skin and coat; in the body, it can be converted to linolenic and arachidonic acids. Linoleic acid deficiency can result in a dull coat, flaking skin, and excessive shedding and scratching. If unsaturated fatty acid deficiency is suspected, add about 1 tablespoon of vegetable oil per pound of dry food or add a food supplement for the skin and coat containing linoleic acid. The symptoms mentioned can have nonnutritional causes; should they persist, seek your veterinarian's advice.

VITAMIN REQUIREMENTS AND DEFICIENCY SIGNS IN THE DOG

Vitamin	Recommended Daily Dietary Level/kg Body Weight Growth	Maintenance	Main Deficiency Sign	Sources	Signs of Hypervitaminosis
A	200 IU	100 IU	Poor growth, xerophthalmia, suppurative skin disease, impaired bone growth	Fish oils, corn, egg yolk, liver	Seen more frequently than deficiency: anorexia, weight loss, decalcification of bone, hyperesthesia, joint ill
D	20 IU (assumes a 1.2:1 calcium: phosphorus ratio)	7 IU	Rickets in young and osteomalacia in adults; also lordosis, chest deformity and poor eruption of permanent teeth	Sunlight, irradiated yeast, fish liver oils, egg yolk	Seen more frequently than deficiency: anorexia, nausea, fatigue, renal damage, soft tissue calcification, hypercalcemia, diarrhea, dehydration, death
E	2.2 mg (depends upon level of unsaturated fat in the ration)	1.1 mg	Reproductive failure with weak or dead fetuses; nutritional muscular dystrophy, steatitis	Egg yolk, corn, milk fat, cereal germs	None recorded
K	Not required except during antibacterial therapy or chronic intestinal diseases		Impaired prothrombin formation, hence reduced clotting time and hemorrhage	Yeast, liver, fish meal, soybeans	None recorded but high levels probably dangerous
C	Not a dietary requirement in normal dogs		Retarded healing, increased susceptibility to disease	Fresh fruits and vegetables; canned orange juice contains about 0.5 mg/ml	Nontoxic
Thiamine	36 mcg	18 mcg	Anorexia, arrested growth, muscular weakness, ataxia	Yeast, liver, whole grains	No toxic effect with moderate overdosage
Riboflavin	.08 mg	.04 mg	Dry scaly skin, erythema of hind legs and chest, muscular weakness in hind quarters, anemia, sudden death	Milk, yeast, and whole grains; dextrin, cornstarch favor synthesis	Nontoxic even in large amounts

Vitamin			Deficiency symptoms	Sources	Toxicity
Niacin	400 mcg	220 mcg	"Black tongue," i.e., anorexia, weight loss, diarrhea, anemia, reddening and ulceration of mucous membranes of mouth and tongue, death	Whole grains, yeast, meat, scraps, tankage, fish meal, eggs; tryptophan for synthesis	Dilation of blood vessels, itching, burning of skin
Pyridoxine	44 mcg	22 mcg	Microcytic hypochromic anemia, high serum iron and atherosclerosis	Whole grains, milk, meat, fish, yeast, liver	No toxicity data has been reported
Pantothenic acid	400 mcg	200 mcg	Anorexia, hypoglycemia, hypochloremia, BUN increase, gastritis, enteritis, convulsions, coma, death	Yeast, dairy products, liver, rice	No data available
Folic acid	8.8 mcg	4.4 mcg	Hypoplasia of bone marrow, hypochromic microcytic anemia, glossitis	Yeast, liver	Nontoxic
Biotin	None on natural diets. Deficiency usually associated with feeding of raw eggs		Tension, aimless wandering, spasticity of hind legs, progressive paralysis	Liver, kidney, milk, egg yolk, yeast	Nontoxic
Cobalamin (B12)	1 mcg	0.7 mcg	Anemia	Liver, fish meal, meat scraps, dairy products	Nontoxic
Choline	55 mg	—	Fatty infiltration of liver, increase in plasma phosphatase, decrease in plasma protein, prothrombin time, hemoglobin and PCV values	Yeast, liver, meat scraps, soybean oil, egg yolk	Persistent diarrhea caused by 10 gms/day or more

Vitamins are necessary for appropriate growth and maintenance of health. They have no caloric or energy value; because they cannot be produced in the body, they must be furnished in the diet. A well-balanced diet, especially a commercially prepared ration, supplies most vitamin requirements. Do not add vitamin supplements to your dog's diet unless they are recommended by a veterinarian to correct specific dietary deficiencies. Food supplements can be beneficial, but an excess of certain vitamins can cause serious problems. An excess of other vitamins, while of no value, is passed out in the urine without producing toxicity.

The fat-soluble vitamins—A, D, E, and K—are indicated in international units (IU), while the water-soluble vitamins—the B-complex group and C—are measured in milligrams and micrograms.

The table* lists vitamin requirements for the dog, their sources, and signs of deficiency or hypervitaminosis.

* Courtesy of Dr. Mark L. Morris, Jr.

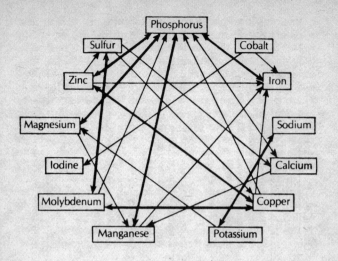

67. MINERAL INTERRELATIONSHIPS

Minerals regulate the chemical balance in the dog's body and act as catalysts for a number of biological reactions. They are components of bones, soft tissues, muscle, teeth, and nerve cells. They help maintain the body's essential fluid balance and the movement of fluids through the cell walls.

Minerals should be considered as a group, since their actions within the dog's body are interrelated. Illus. 67, from *The Collins Guide to Dog Nutrition,* by Dr. Donald R. Collins, shows the interrelationships among minerals. A light arrow indicates that the first mineral is dependent on the second. A bold arrow indicates that they are interdependent.

Because overdose of certain minerals can be harmful, supplementation is not suggested without the advice or recommendation of a veterinarian. The table* lists the mineral requirements of the dog, their sources, and signs of deficiencies.

* Courtesy of Dr. Mark L. Morris, Jr.

MINERAL REQUIREMENTS AND DEFICIENCY SIGNS IN THE DOG

Mineral	Recommended Dietary Level	Sources	Common Deficiency Signs
Calcium	1.0%	Steamed bone meal, dicalcium phosphate, ground green bone, ground oyster shell	Enlarged epiphysis of long bones and ribs, splaying of toes, hyperextension of the carpus and tarsus, spontaneous fractures and abnormal deviation of the legs[a]
Phosphorus	0.9%	Steamed bone meal, dicalcium phosphate, ground green bone	Same as above[a]
Sodium chloride	Not required as such	Table salt	Deficiency is rare. Natural feedstuffs contain adequate amounts. When the deficiency occurs, weight loss, hair loss, acidosis, and eventually death may be seen
Potassium	0.4%	Potassium chloride	Deficiency is rare. Natural foodstuffs contain adequate amounts. When the deficiency occurs, ascending paralysis and depressed reflexes may be seen

[a] Deficiency signs of calcium, phosphorus, vitamin D, magnesium, manganese, or copper may be difficult or impossible to differentiate clinically.

Mineral	Recommended Dietary Level	Sources	Common Deficiency Signs
Magnesium	0.03%	Magnesium carbonate, magnesium oxide, magnesium sulfate	Retarded growth, spreading of toes and hyperextension of carpus and tarsus, hyperirritability, convulsions, soft tissue calcification, enlargement of the epiphysis of long bones[a]
Iron	60 mg/kg of food	Iron carbonate, iron sulfate	Microcytic-hypochromic anemia, anisocytosis and poikilocytosis of erythrocytes
Manganese	5 mg/kg of food	Manganese oxide, manganese carbonate, manganese sulfate	Deficiency is rare. Crooked, shortened soft bones may be seen[a]
Copper	7.3 mg/kg of food	Copper sulfate, copper carbonate, copper oxide	Reduction in erythrocytes, swelling of ends of long-bones, hyperextension of carpus[a]
Zinc	50 mg/kg of food	Zinc oxide	Deficiency is rare. Natural foodstuffs contain adequate amounts except when extreme calcium supplementation is attempted by overzealous dog owners
Iodine	1.5 mg/kg of food	Iodized salt, sodium iodide, potassium iodide	Dead or goitrous pups; erythematous dermatitis

[a] Deficiency, signs of calcium, phosphorus, vitamin D, magnesium, manganese, or copper may be difficult or impossible to differentiate clinically.

343

Water is an essential element in a dog's diet that is often forgotten in discussions of nutrients. A dog can live longer without food than without water. A starving dog can lose up to 40% of its body weight and survive, but a loss of water greater than 15% of normal body weight is fatal.

Your dog should have an adequate supply of fresh drinking water at all times. If access is not free, clean, fresh water should be given three to four times a day. *A dog's water should be of the same quality as what you drink.* How much water a dog consumes depends on several factors:

1. If the dog is a house pet, the type of food it gets is the major factor in determining how much water is necessary. Dry food contains little moisture, and the dog will need more water, either mixed with the food or taken separately. Semimoist and canned foods contain more moisture, but fresh drinking water should still be available
2. Environmental temperature and humidity
3. The dog's temperament and temperature
4. Amount of exercise. *Dogs should not be allowed to drink enormous amounts of water immediately before or after exercise or strenuous activity*

Types of Diets

Most dogs are fed either commercially prepared dog food or homemade diets. Homemade foods (not table scraps) often are given to a dog as its exclusive diet. They can be made with the finest meats, vegetables, and dairy products and be tasty to the dog, but they may not be complete and well-balanced; in addition, they can be expensive and time-consuming. Should you want to feed your dog home-prepared food, a number of recipes for well-balanced diets are suggested in the publications on page 346.

There is such a variety of dog foods to choose from at a supermarket that you may be confused about what to feed your dog. Basically, there are three forms sold: dry, semi- or soft-moist, and canned.

Commercial dry food: Whether served as meal, biscuits, kibble, or expanded particles, dry food is a combination of cereal grains, vegetable products, meat or fish meals, and sometimes dairy products, blended with an appropriate ratio of vitamins and minerals. Most dry foods contain about 10% water, and have a caloric value of 1500 to 1600 calories per pound. Dry food is inexpensive, easy to feed, and convenient to store. Semimoist and canned food is more palatable, but if a dog is given dry food from puppyhood, there should be no problem. Adding a little meat to dry food will heighten palatability.

Semi- or soft-moist food: Semimoist or soft-moist food can be ground (to simulate hamburger), chunk (to simulate frankfurters), or ribboned (to simulate choice cuts of meat). Soybean meal, sugar, meat or meat by-products, animal fat, preservatives, and humectants are blended with an appropriate ratio of vitamins and minerals. Soft-moist foods are usually complete and balanced foods which are palatable, relatively odorless, and convenient to store, requiring no refrigeration. They are easy to feed, being packaged in separately wrapped patties or individual portions in cellophane bags. They contain 25% to 30% water, and deliver 1400 to 1500 digestible calories per pound.

Canned food: This contains 75% to 80% water and delivers 500 to 750 digestible calories per pound; it is usually more palatable and digestible than dry food but is more expensive per pound of dry matter. A pet owner can choose (1) complete, balanced canned foods, a mixture of meat, meat by-products, cereal grains, vegetables, fat, vitamins, and minerals, containing everything the dog needs; (2) canned meats with added vitamins and minerals; and (3) canned meats without added vitamins and minerals. The last two items should be mixed with dry dog food to add taste, not fed as a complete diet.

Special food: A number of foods, such as the Science Diet® line, have been developed to provide optimum nutrition when fed as the sole diet. Each diet is designed for a given life cycle stage or condition: (1) for growing puppies, (2) for pregnancy and lactation, (3) for normal adult dogs, or (4) for stressed or working dogs. The ingredients are 90% digestible and are chosen for biological efficiency, which means that less food is required. The dog uses more of what it eats and the stool waste is only a quarter that of regular dry dog food. Special foods are formulated as a total ration; no supplementation is necessary.

Some dietary foods for dogs with obesity, heart disease, or stomach or intestinal problems, are available in canned and semimoist forms, through your veterinarian.

A high-quality commercially prepared dog food seems to be the best choice. Most of the large commercial manufacturers maintain extensive research facilities for performance studies which help them evaluate and constantly improve their products, which represent the most up-to-date knowledge of nutritional requirements and provide the required nutritional elements in accordance with the recommended minimums for dogs established by the Committee on Animal Nutrition of the National Research Council.

Publications that tell you more about dog nutrition and suggested feeding during the entire life cycle include:

Collins, Donald R.: *The Collins Guide to Dog Nutrition*. Howell Book House, New York, 1972.
Gaines Basic Guide to Canine Nutrition. Gaines Professional Services, White Plains, N.Y., 1977, 4th ed.
McGinnis, Terri: *The Dog and Cat Good Food Book*. Taylor and NG, San Francisco, Calif., 1977.
Morris, Mark L., Jr.: *Canine Dietetics: Nutritional Management in Health and Disease*. Mark Morris Associates, Topeka, Kans., 1977.
National Research Council: *Nutrient Requirements of Dogs*. National Academy of Sciences, Washington, D.C., 1974.

Small dogs require more calories per pound of body weight per day than do large breeds. Adult dogs weighing over 40 pounds require 35 to 40 calories per pound per day, smaller dogs may require 40 to 50 calories per pound per day. However, every dog has its own metabolism and calorie requirements, depending on size, physical condition, amount of activity, and temperature of the environment. If your dog's appetite or weight seems abnormal, seek a veterinarian's advice.

How to Choose a Dog Food

Commercial pet food labeling is carefully controlled by federal and state agencies. The following helpful information appears on all commercial pet food labels:

1. The brand and product name always appear.

2. Information regarding nutritional completeness consists of a statement on whether the food is complete and balanced, containing everything the dog needs, or whether the food is to be used as part of the diet. The Federal Trade Commission has determined that manufacturers cannot make label or advertising claims that a dog food is nutritionally complete or balanced unless it:

(a) Contains ingredients in quantities sufficient to satisfy the estimated nutrient requirements established by a recognized authority on animal nutrition, such as the Committee on Animal Nutrition of the National Research Council of the National Academy of Sciences; or

(b) Contains a combination of ingredients which, when fed to a normal animal as the only source of nourishment, will provide satisfactorily for fertility of the male and female, gestation and lactation, normal growth from weaning to maturity without supplementary feeding and will maintain the normal weight of an adult animal whether working or at rest, and has had its capabilities in this regard demonstrated by adequate testing.

Certain labels may state that the food meets the National Research Council's requirements for the entire life cycle while others may indicate that the food meets the NRC requirements for specific life stages. Read the information to be sure the food meets your pet's needs. If you are confused about label claims, seek your veterinarian's advice.

3. Guaranteed analysis: Generally, a pet food label must list the percentage of *minimum* amount of crude protein and crude fat, and the percentage of *maximum* amount of crude fiber, moisture, and ash. Percentages of minimum amounts of calcium and phosphorus and maximum amounts of salt may be included but are not required by law. The exact amount of specific nutrient is

not given; however, you can get a general idea of the food's contents.

4. List of ingredients: Manufacturers are required to list the ingredients contained in the package in descending order of percentage composition. In *Canine Dietetics*, Dr. Mark L. Morris, Jr., suggests that "by studying the guaranteed analysis, some foods can be eliminated from further consideration. Canned foods that claim a minimum of 3% fat or dry foods with less than 7% fat have such a low caloric density that excessive amounts will have to be consumed to meet the dog's energy requirements. Any canned food containing more than 75% moisture is uneconomical. Also, any food that does not have a guaranteed minimum of at least 0.20% calcium should be eliminated. Any list of ingredients that does not list an animal protein source as one of the first three ingredients, or does not include a cereal grain somewhere in the list, should be eliminated."

5. Net weight of the container: Use this to determine the price per ounce or per pound, which is an important concern for pet owners.

6. The manufacturer's name and address: You can write to seek more information about the food, for example, summaries of feeding studies to verify adequacy claims.

In addition to the label and cost evaluation, Dr. Mark L. Morris, Jr.,* suggests two methods of pet-food screening:

Screening by physical examination. Begin this exam by opening one end of the can and checking for any putrid, rancid, or sour odors. A darkened depression on the surface of the product is not contamination, but an air pocket called the "head space" which aids in creating a vacuum during the canning process. Next open the other end of the can and use the lid to push the contents onto a plate. Using a knife, cut through the food lengthwise (ration-type loaf) or spread a portion on the plate (meat and meat by-products, chunk, or stew products) and attempt to identify the ingredients. A good canned ration food should have a hetero-

* From *Canine Dietetics: Nutritional Management in Health and Disease.*

geneous appearance, containing whole cereal grains and small chunks of animal tissue with no undesirable ingredients (hair, feathers, cereal hulls) or foreign material (sand, wire, paper) evident. A good meat-type food should contain pieces of striated muscle. Large blood vessels, ligaments, tendons, or other connective tissue should not be present: they indicate the presence of inferior quality meat by-products. Examine carefully, as many contain a considerable quantity of textured vegetable protein that appears very similar to pieces of meat.

To evaluate dry foods, check the container for evidence of fat soaking through to the outside, or "grease-out." Dry foods in bags or boxes with "grease-out" occurring are highly susceptible to vermin infestation. Next, take a sample of food from the top and bottom of the bag or box and observe it on a sheet of paper. A great number of tiny particles, or "fines," present in a dry product indicates the food is not one of the better grades. Mold can be detected by odor (musty, stale smell) and by sight (white, blue, green, or black coating on food).

In physically examining soft-moist foods, check the packaging (cellophane wrapper or bag) carefully for any sign of leakage. Soft-moist foods can become contaminated easily if even a small amount of moisture finds its way into the package. A desirable soft-moist product should be free of any off odors or off colors, and feel soft, slightly spongy, and "lubricated" but not wet. Break the soft-moist particle and examine for the presence of cereal by-products. The less desirable products contain considerable quantities of hulls, bran, or cereal wastes.

Feeding trials. Although the price, label, and physical examination provide a great deal of valuable information about a dog food, these factors do not indicate the true nutritional value of the food. The *only* way to be certain of vitamin and trace mineral levels, and protein and fat quality is to feed the food to a dog and observe the results.

Dr. Morris suggests that an easy, short-term test a pet owner can make is to observe the volume of feces produced by a dog. A large quantity of stool generally indicates a poor-quality food; a low level of digestibility is the principal cause of the food's passing unabsorbed into the stool. Another test is whether the food is supplying sufficient energy to support growth or to maintain adult weight. If feeding directions are observed, a food that does not meet this standard should not be fed.

We should add that because balanced, quality foods from large commercial manufacturers are the result of conscientious research, many dogs get a higher level of nutrition from commercial dog foods than their owners get from their own food.

Feeding Methods

The two basic methods of feeding dogs are regulated feeding and self-feeding.

In regulated feeding a specific amount of food is given at fixed times during the day. After weaning, puppies are fed four times a day until they are 3 months of age. From 3 to 6 months of age, they get three meals per day; and after age 6 months, two meals. Most animal nutritionists believe that two daily meals should be continued throughout the pet's lifetime.

Try to give the dog its food at the same times every day, since regularity will help promote a stable appetite and consistent elimination. Regulated feeding also allows you to adjust the amount of food to maintain a stable weight or to promote weight loss or gain. Allow the dog 20 to 30 minutes to eat, then remove the bowl.

In self-feeding the dog has free access to food at all times, eating whatever it wants whenever it wants. This calls for dry or semimoist foods that will remain fresh when left in a dish for hours. Self-feeding has become popular not only with individual owners but with breeding/boarding kennels and veterinary clinics. In the *Gaines® Basic Guide to Canine Nutrition,* it is stated that "self-feeding has many advantages. By eating small amounts on a frequent basis, the level of nutrients in the bloodstream remains more constant. In a clinic or kennel, it has a quieting effect on the dogs and there is no before-mealtime nervous excitement. Being able to nibble at will not only gives the dogs 'something to do' and helps prevent boredom, but generally eliminates coprophagy, or the habit of eating feces. Puppies will usually nibble at the food and not be tempted to investigate stools. Self-feeding has a distinct advantage over 'pack feeding' of a group of puppies or dogs because the less aggressive animals are able to get their share. 'Poor doers' in a kennel generally respond rapidly on such a feeding regimen. . . . This method of feeding has many of the same advantages for the individual pet owner. Since it minimizes boredom, it reduces the chances for the puppy or dog to chew on rugs or furniture and also reduces the worry over not being home for a scheduled feeding."

Convert puppies and older dogs to self-feeding gradually, continuing the regular feeding method for several days but at the same time providing a pan or hopper of dry or soft-moist food at all times. Gradually discontinue the regular feeding in 7 to 10 days, until the dog has adjusted to and accepted self-feeding. Most dogs will consume only the amount of food necessary for their caloric needs, but the one disadvantage to self-feeding is that some dogs overeat and become obese.

Regardless of what feeding method is used, remember to provide clean, fresh drinking water at all times. If free access to water is not possible, it should be offered three to four times daily.

Feeding Suggestions

1. Many pet owners believe that dogs need a variety of foods to satisfy their appetites. Frequent changes in diet are unnecessary and offering a variety of foods often causes digestive disturbances or results in "finicky" eaters. Research has indicated that dogs do best on a single diet and that appetite and weight are less likely to vary when a dog is maintained on the same diet, providing it is complete and balanced.

2. If it is necessary to change a dog's diet, do it over a period of several days to avoid digestive upsets, which while seldom serious or permanent, can involve loss of appetite or diarrhea. To change the diet, on the first day mix one-quarter of the new food with three-quarters of the original diet. The second day, equal parts. The third day, three-quarters of the new diet. The fourth, the new diet.

3. Animal nutritionists do not recommend feeding large amounts of table scraps. The table scraps or people "snacks" fed to a dog tend to be high in fat and carbohydrates and low in protein and calcium. You can give your dog table scraps as treats, or add them to the regular diet in small amounts. Table scraps will not alter a complete and balanced diet if they do not exceed 15% of the dog's daily intake of food.

4. Don't worry if a dog refuses to eat a meal or two. Age, exercise, humidity, or climate can produce a temporary change in a dog's appetite. Unless the condition persists, there is no reason to be apprehensive.

5. If you want to give bones to a dog, be sure they are solid and big enough to be chewed on and not swallowed. Knucklebones and marrow bones are good choices for medium and large breeds. Do not give poultry, steak, chop, or rib bones that can be chewed up and swallowed or can splinter easily, as sharp pieces can become lodged in the throat or pierce the intestinal wall.

6. Try not to let your dog fluctuate in weight. If its appetite or weight is abnormal, seek professional help.

7. Serve the dog's food and water in appropriate bowls. There is a confusing variety of plastic, stainless steel, aluminum, and crockery feeding dishes at pet stores. The bowls should be made of nontoxic material that is easy to clean and dry (and disinfect, if necessary). In addition, feeding dishes should:

a. Not break easily.
b. Not crack, especially if put into a dishwasher or left outdoors in cold weather.
c. Be as "chewproof" as possible, able to withstand abuse from a dog's teeth.
d. Be sturdy enough not to tip over easily or slide across the floor while the dog is eating.
e. If made of plastic, be able to withstand being washed in boiling water without losing shape.

It is also necessary to consider size and shape. It may seem ridiculous, but many pet owners have to be reminded that small dogs should eat from small dishes, medium-sized dogs from medium dishes, and so on. The water bowl should be at least one size larger than the food bowl—perhaps even larger for large and giant breeds or when more than one dog will use it.

Bulldogs, Boxers, Mastiffs, and breeds with similarly shaped heads require wide-bottom feeding dishes, while Spaniels, Poodles, and other long-haired breeds with drop ears should eat from higher, more tapered bowls so that their ears will not hang in the food. Dishes with shallow sides are suggested for Dachshunds and other low-to-the-ground breeds.

8. The same sanitary procedures you use in preparing and serving your meals should be observed for your dog. Food and water bowls should be washed regularly in hot, soapy water and rinsed thoroughly or cleaned in the dishwasher. Food from partly used cans should be transferred to a clean dish, covered with foil or plastic wrap, and refrigerated promptly. Even though soft-moist foods require no refrigeration, when a pouch bag is opened the unused portion should be sealed to keep it from becoming dry and stale. Do not give hot or cold food to the dog; before serving, bring it to room temperature. When canned meat, fresh meat, or a dairy product dish is not eaten (especially in hot weather), it should be picked up after a reasonable amount of time so that the dog does not consume spoiled food.

MISCELLANEOUS PROBLEMS

Flatulence (Gas)

Flatulence, or excessive gas, can occur when a dog is fed a high-protein diet, eats table scraps or highly spiced foods, gobbles its food in large chunks and swallows air, or is overweight or underexercised. Flatulence can also be caused by decomposition of food taken into the body.

This unpleasant condition can often be relieved by changing the diet, or if the dog eats one large meal a day, by separating the daily ration into two or three smaller meals. Try to avoid feeding large quantities of milk or of gas-producing foods like onions, potatoes, beans, and cabbage. Put the pet on regular exercise if necessary.

Feeding activated charcoal tablets after meals may help diminish persistent gas. Consult your veterinarian if this is not successful; he or she may want to prescribe an effective medication or examine the dog to determine if there is an intestinal infection.

Coprophagy (Stool Eating)

Coprophagy, a condition in which a dog eats its own or another animal's stool, is often encountered in puppies and young adult dogs. The exact cause has not been established, but it may be due to bad puppy habits, boredom, or dietary insufficiency. It may be caused by deficiencies of the digestive enzymes amylase, lipase, and protease, causing dogs to eat stools to replace the enzymes.

Stool eating should be discouraged not only because it's repulsive but also, more important, because a dog can acquire internal parasites such as roundworm, hookworm, and whipworm.

If the dog is in good health, discipline and maturity may help break the stool-eating habit. Make sure the dog is properly nourished by a well-balanced diet. Papain, an enzyme found in commercial meat tenderizers, often helps prevent coprophagy. Sprinkle Adolph's, Accent, or some other variety on the dog's food. Use unseasoned meat tenderizer if your dog is prone to gastrointestinal problems; ingredients in the seasoned products may irritate the dog.

20 COMMONSENSE SUGGESTIONS FOR DOG OWNERS

1. Assemble a first-aid kit or buy a preassembled kit. Keep it and a copy of this book in the same location at all times. Make sure that every family member knows where to find it when an emergency occurs.

2. Remember that first aid is not complete treatment, but only emergency action until you can reach a veterinarian. Do not play doctor. Even an insignificant-looking

problem should be checked with a veterinarian. There may be injury or disease that you are not trained to recognize.

3. Become familiar with your dog's normal behavior. When you understand what is normal, you can recognize changes in behavior or general condition that indicate potential trouble.

4. Dogs should have more frequent health examinations than people: they mature almost five times as fast. Your dog should have a general checkup every 6 months.

5. Dogs should be immunized against canine distemper, infectious canine hepatitis, leptospirosis, infectious tracheobronchitis, and rabies. Keep immunizations up to date with the necessary booster shots.

6. Your dog always should wear an identification tag or plate on its collar which gives your name, address, and telephone number. Do not print the dog's name on the tag. Since every dog responds when its name is called, don't give a potential thief this edge.

7. Keep records. In addition to the vital statistics and medical information at the beginning of this section, keep a list of insecticides used on the dog, of food, drugs, and other preparations given to the dog, and of all chemicals used to treat your house or lawn. Someday you may need these records to trace the source of a problem.

8. Before giving a drug, know your dog's weight and the correct dosage.

9. Don't mix drugs; don't use medication that was prescribed for a previous illness. Throw out old drugs and chemicals.

10. Keep your house and yard safe. Inside, keep sharp objects such as sewing supplies, nails, tacks, sharp children's toys, tools, and small bones out of the dog's reach. Keep drugs, chemicals, insecticides, cleaning supplies, paints, varnishes, gasoline, kerosene, plant bulbs, and swimming-pool preparations stored where the dog cannot reach them. (See the lists of potentially dangerous household hazards at "Poisoning" in section I.) Outside, keep the dog away from areas that have been sprayed with insecticides or treated with ant, rat, or snail poison.

11. Before using medications, flea and tick collars, sprays, powders, dips, or other insecticides, read the instructions thoroughly.

12. Do not give your dog chicken, steak, chop, or rib bones that splinter easily, as sharp pieces can become lodged in the throat or pierce the intestinal wall.

13. Do not give a dog, especially a puppy, a toy that can be swallowed whole or torn apart into small pieces and swallowed, possibly causing an intestinal obstruction. Rawhide chips, bones, and chew twists, hard rubber balls and rings, and nylon bones are excellent toys that will be enjoyed by dogs of all ages.

14. Do not allow your dog to run free outdoors. This can result in automobile injuries, poisoning, or bites from other animals. Keep your dog on leash outdoors, especially when you are in a busy or high-traffic area.

15. Don't leave your dog unsupervised in high places from which it can fall, like open windows, rooftops, apartment terraces, balconies or fire escapes, and steep cliffs or hills.

16. Don't allow your dog to ride with its head out the window of a car; exposure to wind and pollution at high speeds can be dangerous.

17. Feed your dog a well-balanced diet, with enough to eat both in quantity and quality for it to be healthy and vigorous. A balanced diet consists of the correct proportions of protein, carbohydrates, fat, vitamins, minerals, and water.

18. Every dog should respond to the five basic obedience commands: "Heel," "Sit," "Come," "Down," and "Stay," and to understand the meaning of the word "No." Obedience training, especially for a pet, helps develop a better understanding between the dog and its owner and encourages the dog's best qualities and behavior. A well-trained dog is welcome almost everywhere. (See "For Additional Reading: Behavior and Training" at the end of the book.) If you find it difficult to train the dog, consider attending classes at an obedience training school where a group of owners are taught how to handle and train their dogs. Most obedience courses consist of 8 to 10 hourly sessions. Owner and dog attend class once a week, practicing for a short time each day at home.

19. Water is an essential nutrient. Every dog should have a supply of clean, fresh drinking water at all times.

20. If your pet will not be bred, consider having it spayed or neutered to prevent accidental breeding. Do

not let your dog carelessly produce unwanted litters of puppies. An altered dog is more gentle and affectionate. Neutered males are less likely to roam, looking for bitches in season. Spayed females will not experience the semiannual heat cycle, requiring confinement to avoid breeding and pregnancy. Altered animals generally live longer. As a male grows older, growths on the testicles and problems with an enlarged prostrate gland are common in unneutered dogs. Unspayed females have a tendency to develop tumors, especially mammary tumors; if these are not removed surgically, they may enlarge, rupture, and become infected or even cancerous.

There is a misconception that altering causes dogs to become fat and inactive. Spaying or neutering has no effect on a dog's weight. Dogs become fat because they eat too much, and inactivity generally accompanies obesity.

The best time to spay a bitch is when she is about 6 months old, before her first heat period. Males should be neutered after they are 6 months old, around the time they begin to raise their legs to urinate. Both operations are relatively uncomplicated; usually, males and females resume normal activities 2 to 3 days after surgery. Spaying or neutering eliminates the sex drive and dogs do not feel or experience sexual desires. They will not feel deprived. Your dog can be spayed or neutered by your veterinarian; but if you cannot afford the full price, low-cost spay-neuter programs are available through many humane shelters or at privately operated spay-neuter clinics.

FOR ADDITIONAL READING

Because of space limitations, books about specific breeds are not included. However, if you own a purebred dog, such books can be invaluable for learning more about your breed.

Behavior and Training

Benjamin, Carole Lea: *Dog Training for Kids*. Howell Book House, New York, 1976.

Fox, Michael W.: *Understanding Your Dog*. Coward, McCann & Geoghegan, New York, 1974. Bantam Books (paper), New York, 1977.

Haggerty, Arthur, and Benjamin, Carole Lea: *Dog Tricks*. Doubleday/Dolphin, New York, 1978.

Koehler, William: *The Koehler Method of Dog Training*. Howell Book House, New York, 1978, 22d printing.

Pearsall, Margaret: *Successful Guide to Dog Training*. Howell Book House, New York, 1976, rev. ed.

Pfaffenberger, Clarence J.: *The New Knowledge of Dog Behavior*. Howell Book House, New York, 1977, 14th printing.

Widmer, Patricia: *Pat Widmer's Dog Training Book*. David McKay, New York, 1977.

Breeding and Reproduction

Harmar, Hilary: *Dogs and How to Breed Them*. T.F.H. Publications, Neptune City, N.J., 1968.

Whitney, Leon: *How to Breed Dogs*. Howell Book House, New York, 1971, rev. ed.

General Care and Information

American Kennel Club: *The Complete Dog Book*. Howell Book House, New York, 1975.

Dangerfield, Stanley, and Howell, Elsworth: *The International Encyclopedia of Dogs*. Howell Book House, New York, 1971.

Denenberg, R. V., and Seidman, Eric: *Dog Catalog.* Grosset & Dunlap, New York, 1978.

Dolensek, Nancy, and Burn, Barbara: *Mutt.* Clarkson N. Potter, New York, 1978.

Harmar, Hilary: *Dogs: Modern Grooming Techniques.* Arco, New York, 1970.

Kalstone, Shirlee: *The Complete Poodle Clipping and Grooming Book.* Howell Book House, New York, 1976, 2d printing.

————: *The Kalstone Guide to Grooming Toy Dogs.* Howell Book House, New York, 1976.

McGinnis, Terri: *The Well Dog Book.* Random House/Bookworks, New York, 1974.

Siegal, Mordecai: *The Good Dog Book.* Macmillan, New York, 1977.

————: *Mordecai Siegal's Happy Pet/Happy Owner Book.* Rawson Associates, New York, 1978.

Stone, Ben, and Migliorini, Mario: *Clipping & Grooming Your Terrier.* Arco, New York, 1970.

————: *Clipping & Grooming Your Spaniel and Setter.* Arco, New York, 1971.

Unkelbach, Kurt: *Best of Breeds Guide for Young Dog Lovers.* G. P. Putnam's Sons, New York, 1978.

Vine, Louis: *Your Dog, His Health and Happiness.* Arco, New York, 1977.

Whitney, George D.: *The Health and Happiness of Your Old Dog.* William Morrow, New York, 1975.

Medical

Kirk, R. W., and Bistner, S. I.: *Handbook of Veterinary Procedures and Emergency Treatment.* W. B. Saunders, Philadelphia, 1975.

Kirk, R. W., et al.: *Current Veterinary Therapy.* W. B. Saunders, Philadelphia, 1976.

Muller, G. H., and Kirk, R. W.: *Small Animal Dermatology.* W. B. Saunders, Philadelphia, 1976.

Pinniger, R. D., ed.: *Jones's Animal Nursing.* Pergamon Press, Oxford, England, 1976, fully rev. 2d ed.

Nutrition

Collins, Donald R.: *The Collins Guide to Dog Nutrition.* Howell Book House, New York, 1972.

Gaines Basic Guide to Canine Nutrition. Gaines Professional Services, White Plains, N.Y., 1977, 4th ed.

Lorenz, Mike, and Morris, Mark L., Jr.: *The G.I. Tract: A*

Commentary on Nutritional Management of Small Animals. Mark Morris Associates, Topeka, Kans., 1976.

McGinnis, Terri: *The Dog and Cat Good Food Book.* Taylor & NG, Brisbane, Calif., 1977.

Morris, Mark L., Jr.: *Canine Dietetics: Nutritional Management in Health and Disease.* Mark Morris Associates, Topeka, Kans., 1977.

Morris, Mark L., Jr., and Teeter, Stanley: *The Guide to Nutritional Management of Small Animals.* Mark Morris Associates, Topeka, Kans., 1976.

INDEX

ABOUT THE AUTHORS

Walter McNamara is the president of a company which produces drugs for pets and is a pioneer in the field of emergency pet care.

Shirlee Kalstone has authored two books on dog grooming and many consumer education booklets on animal health care. Ms. Kalstone also breeds and exhibits whippets and poodles.

Facts at Your Fingertips!

☐ 23595	THE ART OF MIXING DRINKS	$3.50
☐ 23061	EVERYTHING YOU ALWAYS WANTED TO KNOW ABOUT FIRE SAFETY	$2.95
☐ 20832	THE PUBLICITY HANDBOOK	$3.50
☐ 22573	THE BANTAM BOOK OF CORRECT LETTER WRITING	$3.50
☐ 23011	THE COMMON SENSE BOOK OF KITTEN AND CAT CARE	$2.95
☐ 23522	GETTING THINGS DONE	$3.50
☐ 23474	AMY VANDERBILT'S EVERYDAY ETIQUETTE	$3.95
☐ 14954	SOULE'S DICTIONARY OF ENGLISH SYNONYMS	$2.95
☐ 14483	DICTIONARY OF CLASSICAL MYTHOLOGY	$2.75
☐ 14080	THE BETTER HOMES AND GARDENS HANDYMAN BOOK	$3.95
☐ 20085	THE BANTAM NEW COLLEGE SPANISH & ENGLISH DICTIONARY	$2.75
☐ 23111	THE GUINNESS BOOK OF WORLD RECORDS 21st ed.	$3.95
☐ 20957	IT PAYS TO INCREASE YOUR WORD POWER	$2.95
☐ 14890	THE BANTAM COLLEGE FRENCH & ENGLISH DICTIONARY	$2.75
☐ 20298	THE FOOLPROOF GUIDE TO TAKING PICTURES	$3.50
☐ 23393	SCRIBNER/BANTAM ENGLISH DICTIONARY	$2.95
☐ 22975	WRITING AND RESEARCHING TERM PAPERS	$2.95